ESSENTIALS OF FETAL MONITORING

THIRD EDITION

ESSENTIALS OF FETAL MONITORING

THIRD EDITION

By MICHELLE L. MURRAY, PhD, RNC

GAYLE HUELSMANN, BSN, RNC

PATRICIA ROMO, MSN, CNM, RNC

SPRINGER PUBLISHING COMPANY
New York

The information, guidelines, and techniques of practice included in this book are not intended to dictate a plan of care. Publication should not be construed as excluding other acceptable approaches to clinical management. Medication dosages are provided in this book, but it is possible they may change. The reader is urged to review the formulary or manufacturer's package information prior to drug administration.

Springer Publishing Company, LLC
11 West 42nd Street
New York, NY 10036

Acquisitions Editor: James C. Costello
Cover Design: Gaye Roth, Paper Graphiti, Albuquerque, NM
Typeset by: Focus Ink

08 09 10/ 5 4 3

Library of Congress Cataloging-in-Publication Data

Murray, Michelle (Michelle L.) / Essentials of fetal monitoring / by Michelle L. Murray, Gayle Huelsmann, Patricia Romo. — 3rd ed.
p. ; cm.
Includes bibliographical references and index.
ISBN 0-8261-3263-4
1. Fetal heart rate monitoring. 2. Fetal monitoring. I. Huelsmann, Gayle. II. Romo, Patricia. III. Title.
[DNLM: 1. Fetal Monitoring. 2. Heart Rate, Fetal. WQ 209 M983e 2007]

RG628.3.H42M87 2007
618.3'20754--dc22
2006024484

Printed in the United States of America by Bang Printing

"I have found it helpful to recover a sense of my work not as a career but as a calling."

— **D.H. Smith** (June 1994)
"How to Be a Good Doctor in the 1990s: Stand and Deliver"
American Journal of Obstetrics and Gynecology, 170 (6), 1724-1728, p. 1725.

DISCLAIMER

This book is not intended to replace the manufacturer's fetal monitor manual. You are encouraged to read the manual before using the fetal monitor.

This book does not include directions on setting the monitor clock or specific features that are unique to only one or two monitors. Therefore, you are encouraged to work with a skilled clinician who will assist you in setting the clock and using the unique features of your monitor. Since clocks are battery-backed, you should only have to set the clock when there is a change in daylight savings time. If you plug in the monitor and there is a message, e.g., "set time/date," the battery must be replaced. Tag the fetal monitor with a note to replace the clock battery and send it to the Biomedical Department.

Lastly, content of the book is based on references from *Antepartal and Intrapartal Fetal Monitoring, Third Edition* © 2007 and common knowledge in the field of obstetrics and fetal monitoring. Any questions or concerns you have about content should be sent to Springer Publishing Company, LLC.

TABLE OF CONTENTS

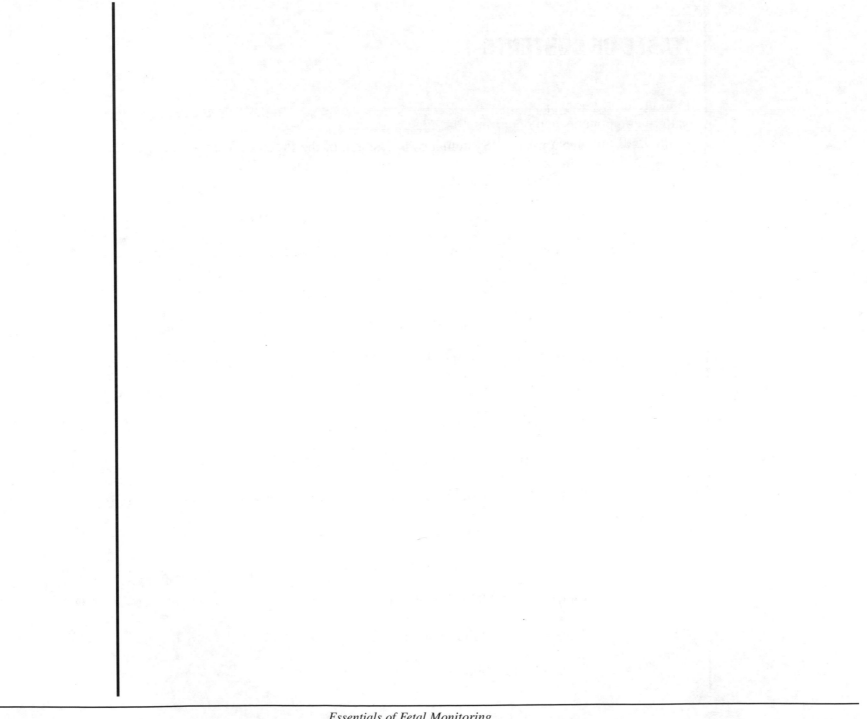

Essentials of Fetal Monitoring

INTRODUCTION

The fetal heart rate (FHR) may be evaluated to predict fetal status. Choosing auscultation or the electronic fetal monitor to evaluate the FHR depends on maternal and fetal risk factors, the nurse to patient ratio, and protocol. If you use the fetal monitor, you will be expected to identify FHR pattern components and determine the significance of the FHR and uterine activity patterns. Although interpretation is subjective, no one can argue with the *absence of any sign of fetal well-being.* Therefore, this book will prepare you to identify the signs of fetal well-being and the more common signs of fetal compromise.

The goals of this workbook are to:
- help you identify maternal and fetal assessment techniques

- prepare you to recognize the most common FHR patterns

- teach you the names of each part of the FHR pattern

- help you select actions to improve fetal oxygenation

- help you evaluate changes in maternal and/or fetal status as a result of your actions

- enable you to identify ineffective actions that delay timely intervention when there is a nonreassuring FHR pattern

- suggest how to document your assessments, actions, evaluations, and communications that reflect the standard of care.

Learning is a journey. This is just the beginning. Knowledge of concepts in fetal monitoring is cumulative. We strongly recommend you plan to attend at least one advanced fetal monitoring course every two years and as many inservice programs as you can to give you more exposure and insight into the fetal condition. Fetal monitors cannot replace hands-on care. They are an adjunct to your care. Therefore, it is important that you touch your patients to palpate contractions and fetal movement.

Michelle L. Murray, PhD, RNC

Trish Romo, MSN, CNM, RNC

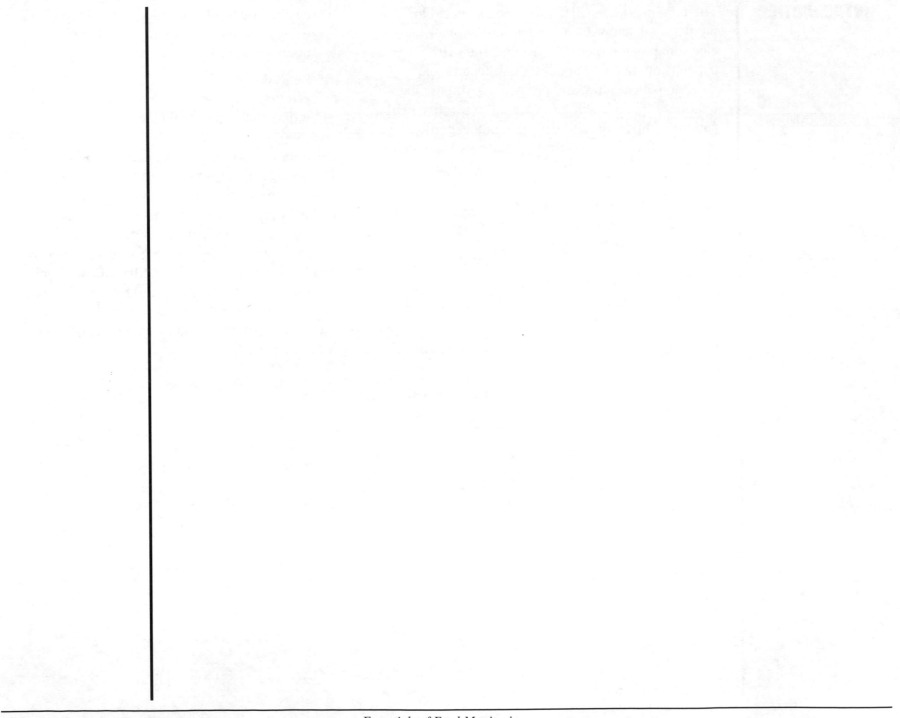

SECTION 1
Systematic Assessment of the Pregnant Woman

The maternal condition affects fetal status. Therefore, it is critical to systematically gather important maternal information prior to interpretation of the fetal heart rate (FHR) pattern. If it is available, review prenatal and historical information prior to approaching the pregnant woman. If the prenatal record is not complete, obtain additional information by interviewing the patient. If possible, obtain a complete prenatal record from the clinic or physician's office. The choice of monitoring methods depends on the practitioner's orders, the institution's policies and procedures, and patient requests or needs. Before approaching the patient, you should know if auscultation and palpation are going to be the only monitoring methods, and if fetal monitoring will be intermittent, continuous, or a combination of both auscultation and electronic fetal monitoring.

Use a systematic approach to evaluate the pregnant woman and fetus. Apply the fetal monitor to complete your assessment of the maternal/fetal dyad. You may choose to do all or part of this assessment prior to monitor use.

Maternal/Fetal Assessment

- Perform Leopold's Maneuvers to locate the fetal back and presenting part
- Estimate fetal weight
- Palpate fetal movement
- Evaluate fetal heart tones by fetoscope
- Assess maternal vital signs and risk factors
- Perform a maternal head to toe assessment
- Determine fundal height – is it appropriate for gestational age?
- Determine uterine activity
- Assess the cervix if there are no contraindications
- Determine the presence of labor and status of membranes

Leopold's Maneuvers

Preparation

Place the woman on her back in a semi-Fowler's position. You may wish to place a pillow under her right hip to displace the uterus off the inferior vena cava and aorta.

You will be inspecting and palpating the maternal abdomen to determine fetal lie and presentation. This will also help you locate the fetal back for external ultrasound transducer placement.

First Maneuver: What is in the Fundus?

Stand at the woman's side and palpate the fundus using both hands. What is in the fundus?

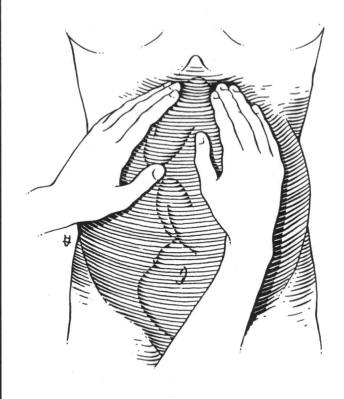

1.1 **First Maneuver - Identify what is in the fundus.** (Reproduced with permission of Appleton & Lange from Oxorn, H. (1986). Human labor and birth, 5th ed. Stanford, CT.)

- *the head feels hard and moves when you push against it*
- *the buttocks feels soft and round*

Second Maneuver: Where is the Fetal Back?

Face the woman and place your hands on either side of her abdomen. While holding one hand still, push on the fetus and feel for the arms and legs and the curve of the fetal back. Now hold the opposite hand still while pushing with the other hand. Can you feel the fetal back? Did the fetus move? You can document fetal movement as "FM palpated" or "FM +." It is very important to keep one hand still so that if the fetus has died you do not mistake pushing the fetus towards the other hand as fetal movement.

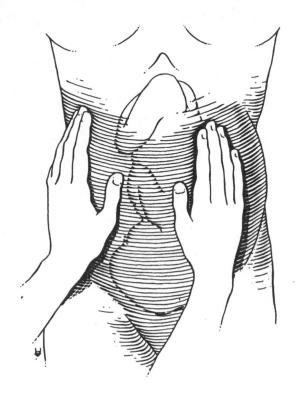

1.2 Second Maneuver - *Find the fetal back.*
(Reproduced with permission of Appleton & Lange from Oxorn, H. (1986). <u>Human labor and birth, 5th ed.</u> Stanford, CT.)

- *the back feels firm, curved, and smooth*
- *the legs, feet, arms, and hands feel irregular*

Third Maneuver: What is the Presenting Part?

Grasp the lower uterine segment by pushing in above the pubic bone. Palpate for a hard or soft mass. If in doubt, the vaginal examination may be helpful to confirm the fetal presenting part.

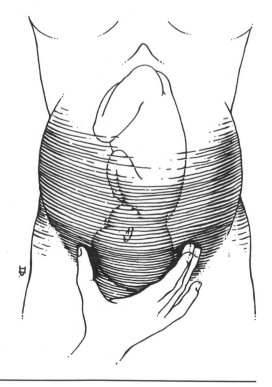

1.3 Third maneuver - *Identify the presenting part.*
(Reproduced with permission of Appleton & Lange from Oxorn, H. (1986). <u>Human labor and birth, 5th ed.</u> Stanford, CT.)

- *the fetal buttocks feels soft and round*
- *the head feels hard and round*

Once you have located the fetal back, what's in the fundus, and the presenting part, you should be able to determine the fetal position. If the back of the baby is on the maternal left (L) side, the occiput (O) is also on the left. The baby will be LOA, LOP, or LOT. The A means anterior, P means posterior, and T means transverse.

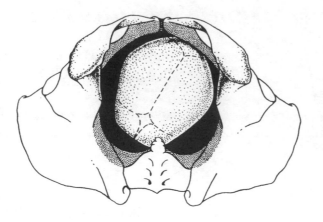

1.4 *This baby is in a left occiput anterior position.* (Reproduced with permission of Appleton & Lange from Oxorn, H. (1986). <u>Human labor and birth, 5th ed.</u> Stanford, CT.)

Fourth Maneuver: Where is the Cephalic Prominence?

When the fetal head is the presenting part, the fourth maneuver will identify the cephalic prominence.

1.5 *Fourth maneuver - Identify the cephalic prominence.* (Reproduced with permission of Appleton & Lange from Oxorn, H. (1986). <u>Human labor and birth, 5th ed.</u> Stanford, CT.)

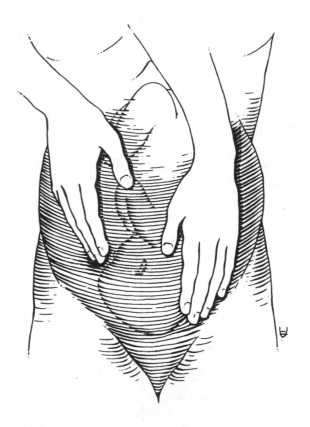

Face the woman's feet and slide your hands down the sides of her uterus until your fingers on one hand meet resistance. This is the cephalic prominence. It may be the baby's forehead or back of the head. If the cephalic prominence is opposite the baby's back, the head is flexed. This is what you want to find. If the occiput is the cephalic prominence, the baby's head is in extension which can impede fetal descent. In this illustration, the fetal forehead is the cephalic prominence.

Estimate the Fetal Weight and Palpate Fetal Movement

When doing Leopold's Maneuvers, you may also estimate the fetal weight. One way to practice is to close your eyes while palpating a 4 pound, 5 pound, and 10 pound sack of sugar which are flat on a table. Feel the difference in the density of the bags. Note the difference between the 4 and 5 pound bag. Is the fetus more like the 5 or 10 pound sack of sugar? As you become more comfortable in estimating fetal weight, it may become easier to predict how well the fetus will fit through the pelvis. Review the maternal obstetric history. Look at the clinical pelvimetry findings in the prenatal record. Does the fundal height suggest a large or small baby? Estimation of fetal weight is important. The risks of fetal macrosomia and fetopelvic disproportion increase with gestational diabetes. Gently place your hand on the maternal abdomen to feel for spontaneous fetal movement.

Evaluate Fetal Heart Rate by Auscultation

Auscultation may be used to intermittently monitor the fetal heart rate, especially in women with no risk factors during labor. Auscultation is not necessary before application of the fetal monitor, but it is desired. **Auscultation confirms fetal life and the FHR.** Before you assess the FHR, confirm the rate from previous monitoring strips or documentation in the prenatal record. For example, a nonstress test result may be written in the prenatal record or the actual FHR may be recorded by the practitioner during prenatal visits. The FHR drops approximately 1 beat per minute (bpm) per week every week of gestation beginning at 9 weeks. The FHR stabilizes at 35 weeks of gestation.

You can confirm fetal life by auscultating fetal heart tones with a fetoscope prior to application of the ultrasound transducer. The FHR can also be determined by a hand-held Doppler device. A fetoscope or stethoscope allows you to hear *tones* or the actual sound of the valves. However, the Doppler is a **motion** detector which determines a *rate*. If a hand-held Doppler is used, it is best to simultaneously assess the maternal pulse to differentiate it from the FHR. Record both the maternal pulse and the FHR. The fetoscope, stethoscope, or Doppler are placed over the fetal back near the baby's head. Listen for at least 30 seconds following a contraction to detect any decelerations. You may want to listen and record a rate every 6 seconds for a full minute. This makes accelerations and decelerations easier to detect. Count the rate for 6 seconds ten times, then add a zero to calculate the beats per minute rates. For example, if you count the first 5 rates for 6 seconds each and record 10, 11, 12, 11, 10, the FHR was 100, 110, 120, 110, and 100. Continue counting for a full minute. In a term or postterm fetus, 100 to 110 bpm is in the normal baseline range.

Confirm Fetal Life

Do **NOT** apply the fetal monitor ultrasound transducer until you are sure the fetus is alive. The printout can be 100% maternal. The woman's heart rate or doubling of her heart rate can appear on the fetal monitor paper (see 1.6). Sometimes, the maternal heart rate (MHR) doubles because the monitor's software analysis counts systole and diastole as two separate beats.

By listening to actual fetal heart sounds with a fetoscope or stethoscope **before** applying the fetal monitor, you can avoid mistaking the MHR for the fetal heart rate. The hand-held Doppler device is a motion, not a sound, detector. If you use a hand-held Doppler device to assess the fetal heart rate, you **must** take the MHR **simultaneously** to identify and differentiate the fetal rate from the maternal rate.

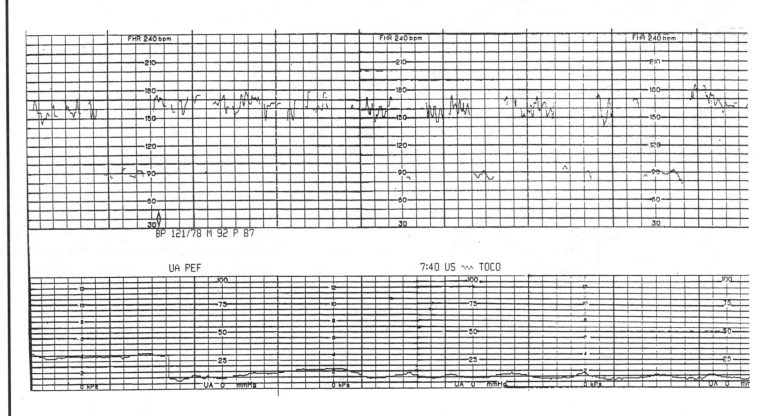

1.6   *Maternal heart rate near 87 beats per minute and doubling near 174 beats per minute. The fetus was dead. The nurse did not confirm fetal life prior to application of the fetal monitor. The lack of fetal heart motion was confirmed by real-time ultrasound.*

Essentials of Fetal Monitoring

Apply the Monitor

To apply the external ultrasound transducer, place the belt under the woman's back. Locate the fetal back. Apply coupling gel to the transducer. Place the transducer over the fetal back. If you have difficulty finding the FHR, move the ultrasound device slightly to the left or right or use the second Leopold's maneuver again to locate the fetal back.

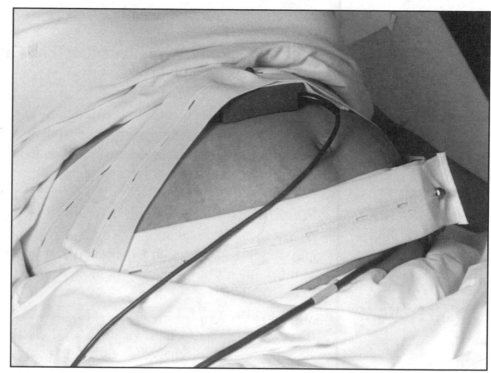

1.7   The ultrasound transducer is placed on the maternal left, over the baby's back and below the umbilicus. The tocotransducer is at the top of the uterus.

FETAL WELL-BEING

The presence of a stable FHR, an acceleration, and the absence of a deceleration, during the period of time the patient is auscultated suggests fetal well-being. The lack of fetal well-being requires prompt communication. *Prompt communication to the midwife or physician about changes in the maternal or fetal status is the nurse's role.*

Auscultation can be used during labor when a one-to-one nurse to patient ratio is available. Documentation should include the presence of accelerations, the absence or presence of decelerations, and the FHR between accelerations and decelerations. For example, you might mention "no decelerations heard." Also, document any fetal movement (FM) palpated or reported, e.g., "fetus active per pt., FM palpated."

Auscultation: Abnormal Findings

A FHR greater than 160 bpm, less than 120 bpm if the fetus is preterm, and less than 100 bpm if the fetus is term or post term, or an irregular rhythm should be reported to the midwife or physician as soon as possible. Also, report any FHR which is greater than 20 bpm above or below the baby's expected rate based on previous monitoring. Apply the electronic fetal monitor if you hear a rate greater than 160, less than 100 in a term or post term pregnancy, less than 120 in a preterm pregnancy, or an irregular rhythm.

Assess Maternal Vital Signs and Risk Factors

Take the woman's blood pressure (BP) and pulse. The cuff must be an appropriate size and should be approximately 20% wider than the width of her arm. The woman should have her BP taken in a semi-Fowler's or side-lying position versus supine. It is best to take BP between contractions because BP rises during contractions. Compare the readings with the woman's baseline BP on her prenatal record. If the BP is elevated, pay special attention to her urine protein, edema, and reflexes. Also assess visual disturbances, headache, and epigastric pain. Could she have preeclampsia?

Respiratory Rate

Assess maternal respirations. Are they rapid and labored? Quiet and slow? An unusually fast rate (> 24/minute) may suggest anxiety with hyperventilation or a compromised respiratory system requiring further assessment of the woman's pulmonary or hemodynamic status and temperature.

Temperature

If the woman's temperature is elevated, look for signs of infection such as skin that is warm to the touch, foul smelling vaginal discharge, a tender uterus, fetal tachycardia (> 160 bpm), and/or maternal tachycardia (> 100 bpm). Assess skin turgor, mucous membranes, and lips for dryness. If she is febrile, she may also be dehydrated. Assess her urine for ketones.

HEAD TO TOE ASSESSMENT

Perform a Maternal Head to Toe Assessment

	FINDINGS
HEENT (head, eyes, ears, nose, and throat)	headache, blurred vision, tinnitus, nasal congestion, airway, dizziness?
Heart	regular rate and rhythm, murmur, chest pain, palpitations?
Lungs	clear breath sounds bilaterally, unlabored respirations? absence of wheezing, grunting, adventitious sounds?
Abdomen	tenderness, pain, rigidity, distention, heartburn? quality and quantity of contractions? fetal movement?
Extremities	edema, reflexes, clonus? Homan's sign?
Genitourinary	urine protein, ketones, glucose, blood? genital vesicles or warts? rupture of membranes?

COMPLETING YOUR ASSESSMENT

Inspection, palpation, and auscultation are used to complete your initial maternal assessment. Observe the woman's general appearance and body language which provide clues of underlying physical or psychological problems. Ask when she last ate and what she ate. When she is alone, ask if she has been hit, slapped, kicked, or punched any time during this pregnancy. Ascertain if she has had any bleeding problems, a history of previous hemorrhage with birth, or blood transfusions. This may prepare you for the possibility of a postpartum hemorrhage or a newborn with hemolysis as a result of an antibody-antigen reaction. Record your findings. Ask her to urinate prior to her cervical examination. A sterile speculum examination may be done to prevent infection if membranes are ruptured, but she is not in labor.

FUNDAL HEIGHT AND FETAL GROWTH

Determine Fundal Height — Is it Appropriate for Gestational Age?

What is the estimated date of delivery (EDD)? If fundal height has not been measured in the last week, or you are concerned that the placenta may be abrupting, measure the fundal height by placing a tape measure at the top of the symphysis pubis, and stretch it to the top of the fundus. Mark the top of the fundus using a ballpoint pen if you plan to measure and compare findings at a later time.

After the 20th week of pregnancy, the fundal height is similar to the weeks of gestation. If there is a 3 or more centimeter difference, e.g., she is 26 weeks of gestation, but the fundal height is 23 centimeters (cm) or 29 cm, an ultrasound may be done to identify an abnormality in fetal growth or amniotic fluid volume.

When the fundal height is smaller than expected (not within 3 cm of the gestational age), review the prenatal history for persistent vomiting, poor weight gain, hypertension, street drug use, and smoking. These could diminish oxygen and nutrient delivery to the uterus. Hydramnios, macrosomia, a fibroid, and gestational diabetes may be associated with a larger than expected fundal height, and oligohydramnios and/or intrauterine growth restriction with a smaller than expected fundal height.

UTERINE ACTIVITY

Determine Uterine Activity

Palpate the woman's uterus. Assess the symmetry of the abdomen during contractions. During normal labor, the uterus begins to contract at the fundus and the fundus moves forward. Record "mild," "moderate," or "strong" uterine contractions. If some are mild and others are moderate, record "UCs mild–mod" or "ctx mild to mod." Feel your cheek. It's indentable. That's how a mild contraction feels. Feel your nose. A little harder, but slightly indentable is how a moderate contraction feels. Feel your forehead. This is how a strong contraction feels to palpation.

LABOR

Determine the Presence of Labor and Status of Membranes

Labor is defined as regular uterine contractions accompanied by a change in dilatation. Determine the presence of contractions. Evaluate maternal pain by observing the woman's face, hands, and toes. Is she curling her toes or tightening her grasp? Perhaps she is focused inwardly, suggesting advanced labor progress. Is her pain response what you would anticipate with the contractions you palpate? What impact does her culture have on her display of pain? Nitrazine paper or a Fern test may detect rupture of membranes. If membranes are ruptured, record the color, amount, and odor of the fluid (**1 milliliter (ml) of fluid weighs 1 gram (gm)**). Determine if there is a vaginal discharge or foul odor. The odor may be recorded as "foul" or "not foul."

Essentials of Fetal Monitoring

Prior to applying the fetal monitor

- assess comfort or pain, readiness to learn, and previous experiences with the fetal monitor

- address concerns about the electronic fetal monitor (EFM), explain the monitor's function and plans for use

- adapt the monitoring belts if needed for the obese patient, e.g., attach one belt to another one or hand-hold the ultrasound transducer

- do not use the ultrasound transducer or spiral electrode if the fetus is not viable (≤ 23 weeks) or has died

- do not apply the monitor if the woman refuses it.

If a women refuses electronic fetal monitor use, the physician or midwife should be informed immediately. Document the patient's refusal by recording her words in quotation marks.

PLACEMENT OF THE TOCO-TRANSDUCER

Secure the tocotransducer (TOCO). Correct placement of the TOCO should detect uterine contractions not maternal breathing movements. The TOCO works best close to term. If the fetus is less than 30 weeks of gestation, place the TOCO under the umbilicus. Ask the woman is she has cramps, intermittent bladder pressure, intermittent leg pain or low backache. These may be indications of preterm labor. Place the TOCO above the umbilicus if the fetus is greater than 30 weeks of gestation (see 1.9).

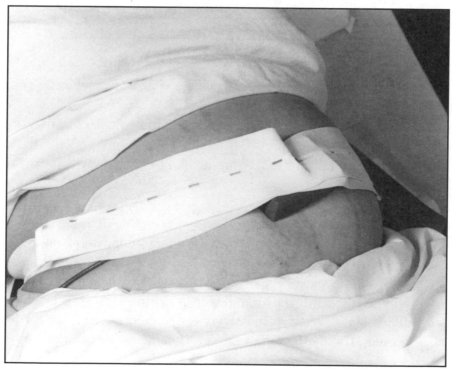

1.8   Preterm pregnancy tocotransducer placement.

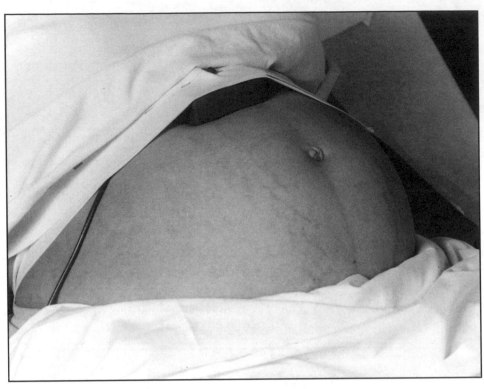

1.9   ***Term pregnancy tocotransducer placement.***

THE CERVIX

Assess the Cervix

Defer cervical examinations when bleeding is present until you know the location of the placenta, e.g., avoid a vaginal examination if there is placenta previa. If membranes rupture preterm, the cervix may be examined visually using a sterile speculum. This prevents introduction of bacteria which can stimulate prostaglandin release and contractions.

During cervical examination, assess
- location   locate the cervical os. Is it posterior, in a midposition, or anterior?

- dilatation   estimate the size of the opening of the cervix in centimeters using your index and middle fingers. If only one fingertip fits inside, it is "FT" or fingertip dilated. This is equivalent to 1 cm. If the cervix is open more than 9 cm but less than 10 cm, a "rim" is present. If only the top of the cervix remains, an anterior lip ("ant. lip") is documented.

- effacement

  how thin is the cervix? At term, the cervix is approximately 2.5 to 3 cm long. It may be firm or soft. Effacement occurs when the cervix is soft. It is estimated as the percent that has thinned, e.g. 70% effaced means only 30% remains.

- presentation

  vertex, breech, or other, e.g., face, brow, shoulder. Is there caput or molding? cord or compound presentation, e.g., head and hand?

- station

  determine the level of the presenting part above or below the ischial spines. When the tip of the baby's skull is at the level of the ischial spines, that is zero (0) station. Use centimeters: -1, -2, -3, ballottable (all are above the spines), +1, +2, +3, +4, +5 (are below the spines).

SUMMARY

Summary

Establish a data base that includes maternal, FHR, and fetal movement information. Continue to evaluate the woman and fetus. Once the plan of care is determined, the midwife or physician usually discusses the plan with the woman and her family. Assessment of her initial and ongoing status and behavior may reflect normal or abnormal progress which may influence the FHR. *Always try to respond to maternal and fetal physiology.* It can affect the FHR. Think beyond the paper printout and "know the baby."

SECTION 1: SYSTEMATIC ASSESSMENT OF THE PREGNANT WOMAN

QUESTIONS

Directions: Circle T if the statement is true, F if it is false.

QUESTIONS

T	F	1. A systematic assessment of the pregnant woman includes Leopold's Maneuvers.
T	F	2. The choice of monitoring methods depends on the number of registered nurses and patients.
T	F	3. Auscultation of fetal heart tones is desired prior to application of the fetal monitor.
T	F	4. When a fetoscope is used, document the fetal heart rate, accelerations, and decelerations.
T	F	5. The initial assessment may include fundal height to rule out intrauterine growth restriction or fetal macrosomia.
T	F	6. A cervical examination can confirm the fetal presenting part.
T	F	7. At 26 weeks of gestation, the tocotransducer should be placed above the umbilicus.
T	F	8. It is important to consider the impact of maternal and fetal physiology on the FHR.

SECTION 2
The Paper

STRIP OR TRACING

You may recall from Section 1 that it is best to observe and respond to the fetal and maternal physiology that produces the FHR printout. The printout is also called a *strip or tracing*.

PAPER SPEED

In the United States, the tracing flows out of the fetal monitor at 3 centimeters (cm) per minute. In some countries this speed is reduced to 1 or 2 cm/minute. In the United States the paper speed standard is 3 cm/minute. **Find the paper speed switch on your fetal monitor.** If it is set at 1 or 2 cm/minute, the image will be compressed and may be misinterpreted. Change it to 3 cm/minute.

HEAT-SENSITIVE PAPER

The tracing is printed on *heat-sensitive* paper. It turns black when a hot printer touches it. The paper is printed with two channels. The upper portion or fetal heart rate channel is 30 to 240 beats per minute (bpm) or 50 to 210 bpm. The lower portion or uterine activity (UA) channel is usually 0 to 100 mm Hg or 0 to 90 mm Hg.

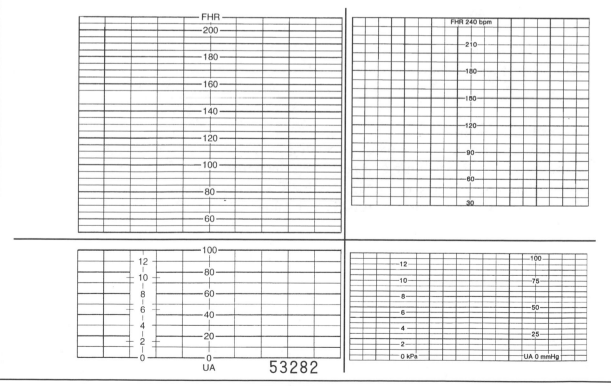

2.1
The fetal heart rate channel is always at the top of fetal monitoring paper and the uterine activity channel is at the bottom.

INK

The color of the grid on the paper is *not* significant. What is important is the numeric scale on the FHR channel.

USA SCALE PAPER

Look again at the fetal heart rate channel on the paper on the right. It is 30 to 240 bpm. Each ascending horizontal line is 10 bpm above the line below it. This is called USA scale paper.

EUROPEAN SCALE PAPER

The fetal heart rate channel on the paper on the left is 50 to 210 bpm and each ascending horizontal line is 5 bpm above the line below it. This is called European scale or International scale paper, to differentiate it from USA scale paper. Some European scale paper has a range of 60 to 200 bpm. Both types of paper may be used in any fetal monitor *provided the machine is adjusted to print on that scale.*

REVIEW QUESTION

All fetal monitor paper, whether USA or International scale, should roll out of the electronic fetal monitor at the same speed. What is that speed in the United States?

If you said 3 cm/minute you're right! Now look again at the USA scale fetal monitor paper. Notice the vertical lines on the FHR channel. As your eye moves from left to right, count 6 small squares. Each square is 10 seconds in duration. Six squares are equal to one minute of time. Each minute is 3 cm in length. The paper on the left has 20 seconds between each vertical line. On both types of paper, 1 cm equals 20 seconds and 3 cm equals 1 minute.

Whether or not you have European or USA scale paper in the machine, it should be moving out of the fetal monitor at 3 cm/minute. If your hospital changes from USA to European scale paper or vice versa, a biomedical technician must adjust the fetal monitor printer or the printed image of the FHR will be inaccurate.

LOADING THE PAPER

Loading the Paper

When you load the fetal monitor paper, the *FHR* channel should be on the *left* and the UA channel will be on the *right*. **Practice loading and removing the paper**. Read the directions on the paper package and follow the guidelines. Some paper loads with the first sheet on the bottom of the paper pack. Each paper pack lasts at least 8 hours when the paper speed is 3 cm/minute.

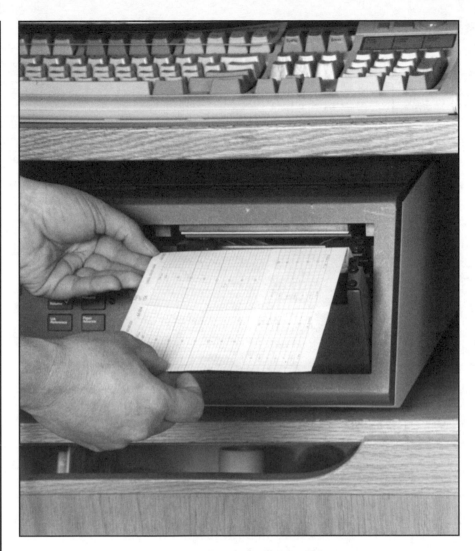

2.2 *When the fetal monitor paper is loaded properly, the FHR will print on the channel on the left and uterine activity will print on the channel on the right.*
(Photograph by Pam Barncastle, Castle Studio, Albuquerque, New Mexico).

DOCUMENTATION

Documentation When You Begin Monitoring

Your facility may have a specific policy on what should be written on the first square of the fetal monitor paper. If not, it is best to write patient identifying information. If the fetal monitor does not print the date on the tracing and the monitoring start time, it should be written. Any additional information, e.g., the admitting practitioner, may be added to help identify this legal document.

Strip with Initial Documentation

```
07:56    3 CM/M  HR1:US
12/06/95  UA:EXT  HR2:OUT
```

#1
Doe, Jane 1234567
$G_2 P_0$
Dr./CNM Patience
EDD 12/8/2001

test lines

2.3   Label the tracing with patient identifying information and the number of the strip. Also note lines are printed as a monitor/printer test when the monitoring begins. See test lines.

NUMBER THE TRACING

Number 1 signifies this is the first tracing generated in Jane Doe's visit. If for any reason the tracing is torn off (pages are perforated), or the paper is changed, each consecutive tracing should be numbered, e.g., #2, #3. This helps put the tracings in consecutive order before they are submitted to Medical Records.

Initial labeling should include the woman's name and medical record number, how many times she has been pregnant (gravida "G"), the number of babies delivered who weighed at least 500 grams or who had a gestational age of 20 weeks or more (one definition of parity "P"), her physician or midwife's name, and her estimated date of delivery at 40 weeks of gestation. Record the same information on consecutive strips.

Testing the Fetal Monitor

Now that the paper is in the machine and it is properly labeled, turn the fetal monitor on. Be sure the paper is moving. Is the record button on? The **auto test** feature should be automatically activated. The printer will print and the digital display will be illuminated. Look at the lines printed on the paper as the paper advances. There should be no gaps. Look at the lighted display. Are the numbers totally illuminated? If there are gaps on the test lines or if the printer is not printing on the paper lines, the printer needs to be repaired or perhaps the paper feed needs to be adjusted. Tag the fetal monitor "printer not properly printing," include a sample of the misprinted paper, and send the monitor to the Biomedical Department.

If you wish to see the test strip again, or if the monitor does not perform an auto test, push the **test** button for a **manual test** to document that the monitor printer was properly functioning prior to use.

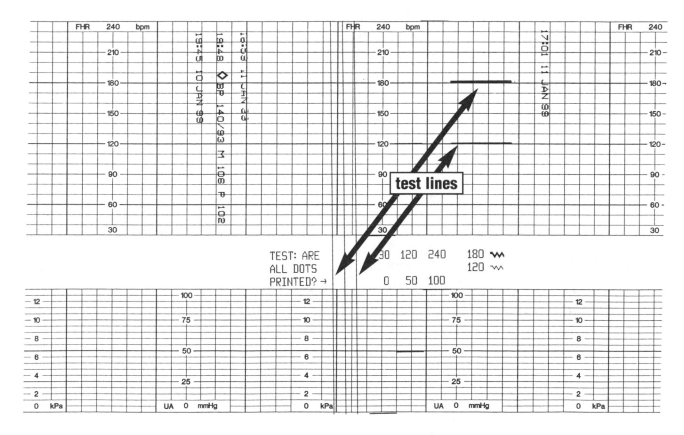

2.4   All the printed lines should be continuous and on the paper lines. If the test lines are not on the paper lines, the printer or paper feed needs to be adjusted by biomedical personnel.

You can also test each internal and external FHR and uterine activity component that plugs into the fetal monitor. These specific tests will be discussed in Section 3: External and Internal Fetal Monitoring.

THE CLOCK

A battery backs up the monitor clock so that even when it is unplugged the date and time will remain set. If you plug in and turn on the fetal monitor, and a message is printed on the paper stating "set time/date," the battery is dead. Label the fetal monitor with a note, "replace clock battery" and send the monitor to the Biomedical Department or ask them to replace the battery at the fetal monitor location.

Learn how to set the time and date. All monitors should be set to the same time. First, set one watch to the main operating room clock. Then, each monitor clock is set using that watch. Set your watch to the monitor time so that when you care for more than one woman, documented events will reflect the time on all the fetal monitors.

EXERCISES

EXERCISES

1. What is the FHR range of USA scale paper?
   a. 50 to 210 bpm
   b. 30 to 240 bpm
   c. 30 to 200 bpm

2. What is the FHR range of most International scale paper?
   a. 50 to 210 bpm
   b. 30 to 240 bpm
   c. 30 to 200 bpm

3. What is the paper speed in the United States?
   a. 1 cm/minute
   b. 2 cm/minute
   c. 3 cm/minute

4. What does it mean when the print-out on the paper is "set time/date?"
   a. the time is wrong and needs to be reset
   b. the clock back-up battery needs to be replaced
   c. this message always appears when the monitor is turned on

5. Which of the following is not needed when the fetal monitor is initiated?
   a. woman's name
   b. identification number
   c. maternal diagnosis

See page 29 for the correct responses.

Maternal Heart Rate (MHR)

Since women have variability or fluctuations of their heart rate it is possible that the MHR will print when the fetus has died or the external ultrasound transducer is over the maternal aorta. By comparing maternal pulse **simultaneously** with the printed rate, you should be able to confirm that you are not recording the MHR. If you are concerned, confirm the fetal heart rate by listening to fetal heart sounds with a fetoscope or apply the fetal monitor's **maternal 3-lead ECG cable** (see figure 2.5) or pulse oximeter (see 2.6) to obtain a continous MHR printout on the tracing. You can also apply a free-standing pulse oximeter and compare the pulsation sound with sound generated by the fetal monitor. They should differ. If the MHR and printout coincide, the FHR is not being recorded. Use a fetoscope or real-time ultrasound to confirm fetal cardiac motion and the FHR.

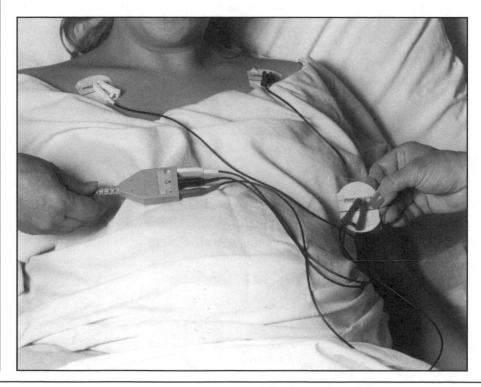

2.5 ***Maternal 3 lead ECG cable for the fetal monitor.***
(Photograph by Pam Barncastle, Castle Studio, Albuquerque, New Mexico).

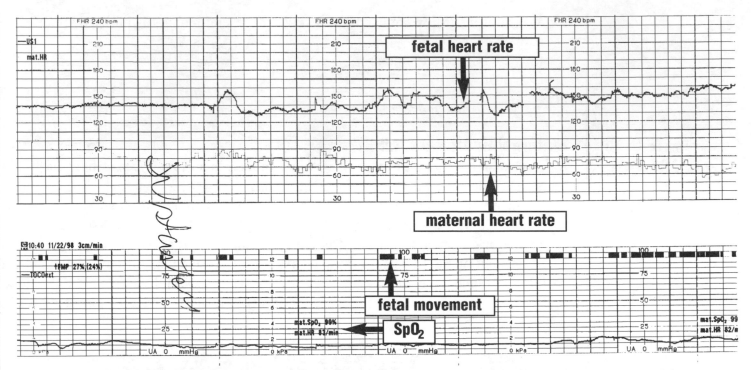

2.6   *Fetal heart rate demonstrating fetal well-being. The baseline is initially near 140 bpm with spontaneous accelerations. Maternal heart rate assessed by the pulse oximeter is 65-80 bpm. Note there is variability. Fetal movement is indicated by black marks on the top of the uterine activity channel and maternal SpO$_2$ is 99%.*

TWIN MONITORING

Twin Monitoring

Two ultrasound transducers may record the same fetus when both are directed towards one fetus or the spiral electrode (internal monitor) and ultrasound (external monitor) are on the same fetus. Depending on the manufacturer, there may be an indication this is happening, e.g., Hewlett Packard series 50 monitors will print a ? on the top of the FHR channel. This is called **cross-channel verification** (see 2.7). If this occurs, locate the other fetus by palpation and reposition the ultrasound. A fetoscope or real-time ultrasound may be needed to confirm fetal life.

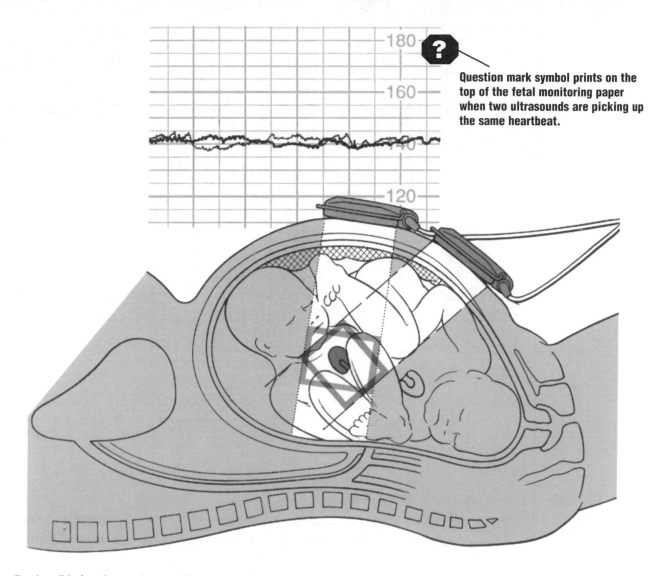

Question mark symbol prints on the top of the fetal monitoring paper when two ultrasounds are picking up the same heartbeat.

2.7   Series 50 fetal monitor with cross-channel verification (provided with permission of Hewlett-Packard® Company).

BASELINE OFFSET

Sometimes the fetuses are clearly recorded but the FHR patterns are in the same range, making it difficult to see each FHR. By pushing a button, e.g., the *mark* button on the *Corometrics*® 116, 118, or 120 series monitors, the twins will be separated by 20 bpm. This is called a **baseline offset**. The baseline offset of the Spacelabs fetal monitor is 30 bpm. *Toitu*® monitors label each fetus and each fetus' activity (see book cover).

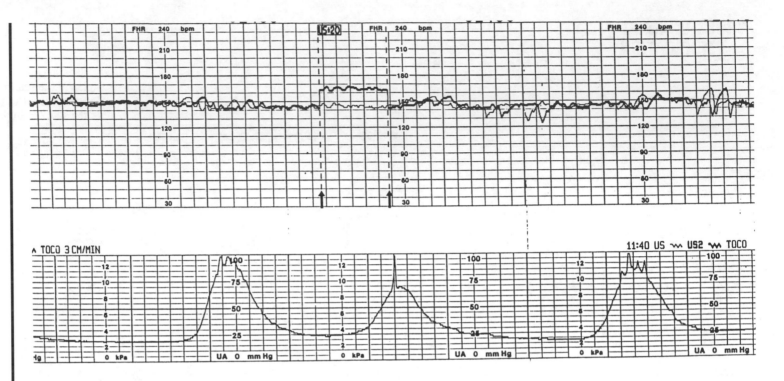

2.8 *Baseline offset of Corometrics® fetal monitor. Pushing the mark button for 3 seconds elevates one twin's rate. Pushing the mark button again returns it to its normal level.*

Documentation of Twins

If you are not sure that both twins are alive, listen for two different heart rates using a fetoscope or ask the appropriately skilled clinician to assess fetal cardiac motion using a real-time ultrasound machine.

When you begin monitoring, label each respective tracing "Twin A" and "Twin B." This can be repeated from time to time, e.g., every half hour to hour. If twin B delivers first, the note on the delivery summary should read "First twin (B), second twin (A)." If you are performing an antepartal test, such as a nonstress test, note twin A's and Twin B's average heart rate in the prenatal record. Try to keep A as A and B as B in subsequent monitoring. The FHR drops approximately 1 bpm per week of gestation beginning at 9 to 10 weeks of gestation. The FHR stabilizes at 35 weeks. If each twin has a different average FHR, e.g., 130 bpm and 150 bpm, it should be easy to keep them as A and B throughout the pregnancy.

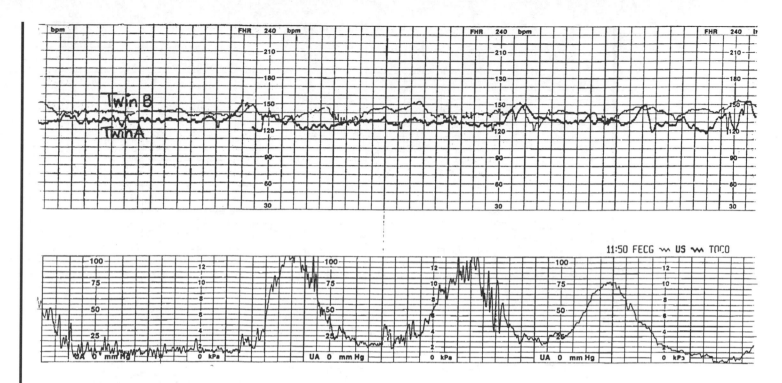

2.9 *Label the FHR of each twin every $^1/_2$ to 1 hour. This helps anyone who reviews the strip easily verify fetal status.*

Maternal Heart Rate Doubling and Fetal Heart Rate Halving

The maternal heart rate will be recorded when the fetus is dead or the ultrasound transducer is over the maternal aorta. The maternal heart rate may double, but only when the ultrasound transducer is used. The actual maternal heart rate is printed (no doubling) when a spiral electrode is on the fetus. The fetal heart rate **never** doubles with second-generation monitors. However, if the fetal heart rate exceeds the paper scale, it will halve, e.g., a rate of 300 bpm will print at 150 bpm. This occurs when the fetus has supraventricular tachycardia.

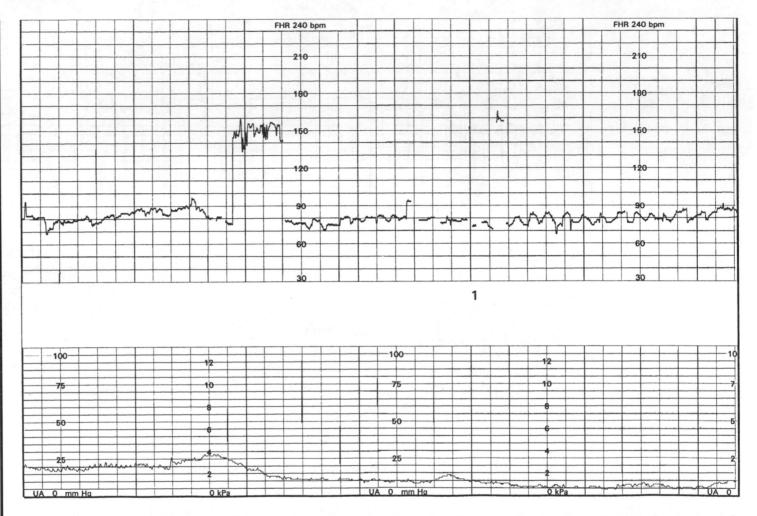

2.10 *Doubling of the maternal heart rate can occur when the ultrasound transducer is over the maternal aorta. However, second-generation fetal monitors **never** double the fetal heart rate. Most monitors created in the 1980s and beyond are second-generation monitors.*

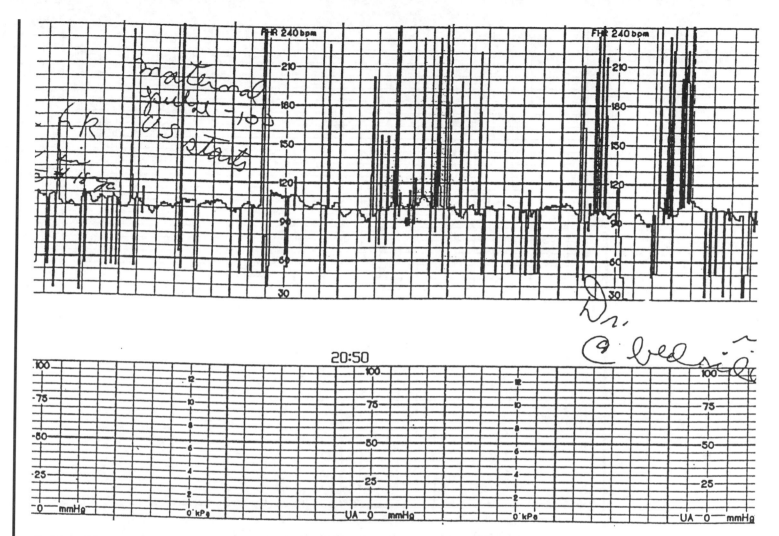

2.11   *The maternal heart rate averages 100 bpm in this tracing. A spiral electrode was on the fetus who was dead and it transmitted the maternal ECG signal into the fetal monitor where the bpm rate was calculated then printed. Note artifact lines. Artifact is due to signal interruption.*

Healthy women have short-term and long-term variability. When a spiral electrode is on the fetus, artifact appears as vertical lines of various lengths. Artifact is caused by interruption of the signal through the spiral electrode. Be sure to confirm fetal life before the fetal monitor is applied.

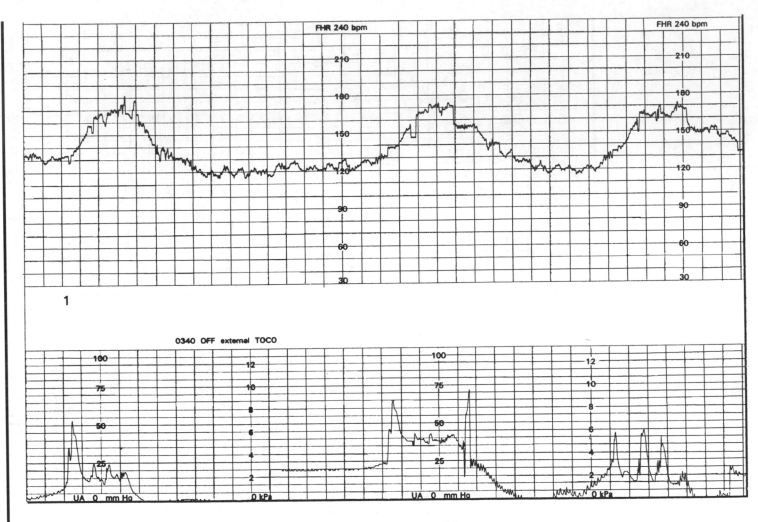

2.12   Maternal heart rate accelerations with pain during pushing.

The maternal heart rate will accelerate in response to pain, especially during pushing. Sometimes the maternal heart rate decelerates during contractions.

ANSWERS TO EXERCISES

1. b
2. a
3. c
4. b
5. c

SUMMARY

Summary

USA scale paper has a range of 30 to 240 bpm. Each ascending horizontal line is 10 bpm higher than the line below it. Usually the paper is printed in 10 second blocks with each square moving from left to right representing 10 seconds of time. Thus, six boxes represent a minute of time. The paper speed is 3 cm/minute in the United States. Confirm fetal life then apply the monitor. When using a fetal monitor start by testing it. Label the fetal heart rate tracing with identifying information. Determine if the tracing represents a maternal or fetal heart rate by comparing the printout simultaneously with the maternal pulse or printout from the pulse oximeter or maternal 3-lead ECG. If the rate is maternal, locate the fetal back, reapply gel to the ultrasound transducer if needed, and place the transducer over the fetal heart. Label twins on the monitor tracing as Twin A and Twin B every $1/2$ to 1 hour. If twin B is delivered first, identification bands should list "1st twin (B)."

SECTION 2: THE PAPER

QUESTIONS

Directions: Circle T if the statement is true, F if it is false.

QUESTIONS

T F	1.	International scale paper speed is 1 cm/minute.
T F	2.	On USA scale paper, each 20 seconds equals 1 cm in length.
T F	3.	If the paper is loaded correctly, the fetal heart rate channel is on the right.
T F	4.	Parity has been defined as the number of live babies delivered after 20 weeks of gestation.
T F	5.	It is acceptable to use a fetal monitor even if the printer test strip lines are misaligned with the paper grid.
T F	6.	The maternal heart rate can print on the fetal monitor paper.
T F	7.	If twin B delivers first, the baby becomes twin A.
T F	8.	Fetal heart rates can double with second-generation monitors.
T F	9.	The maternal pain response may cause accelerations of the maternal heart rate.
T F	10.	The maternal heart rate may decelerate.

SECTION 3
External and Internal Fetal Monitoring

ULTRASOUND TECHNOLOGY: EXTERNAL FHR MONITORING

Peak Detection

Fetal monitors have changed over the last thirty years. You are probably not using fetal monitors made in the 1970s and early 1980s. The first generation monitors determined the fetal heart rate (FHR) by detection of the ultrasound waveform peaks, thought to represent systole of the heartbeat. The beat-to-beat interval was estimated. A beats per minute (bpm) rate was determined and was printed. Some of the old sayings when these monitors were used were:

- *"If it looks bad on external, it's worse on internal."* (meaning the ultrasound tracing that looked nearly smooth, would be even smoother when a spiral electrode was used)
- *"Don't document beat-to-beat variability when an external is used."* (meaning the printout generated with an external ultrasound may be bumpy; while the printout from a spiral electrode is smooth)

Autocorrelation

The change and improvement in ultrasound hardware and software in the 1980s improved analysis of the ultrasound signal. The new software uses a process called autocorrelation to analyze the ultrasound waveform created by the movement of the heart, the heart valves, and even the fetus. Monitors that use autocorrelation are called second-generation monitors. With autocorrelation, the printed rate is within 2.5 bpm of the true rate. A high-speed data processor analyzes each incoming nonrandom ultrasound signal generated by fetal mitral and tricuspid valve movement. After 0.5 to 1.2 seconds are analyzed, the FHR is calculated and printed. The printed rates, when connected, create a FHR baseline, accelerations, and decelerations.

Ultrasound (US) Principles

- The US detects movement, not electrical energy or sound.
- Movement of the heart valves creates US waveforms for counting.
- Analysis of the US signal depends on the software capabilities of the fetal monitor.
- **Little additional clinical information will be gained by the application of a spiral electrode when compared with a consistent ultrasound-derived FHR pattern.**

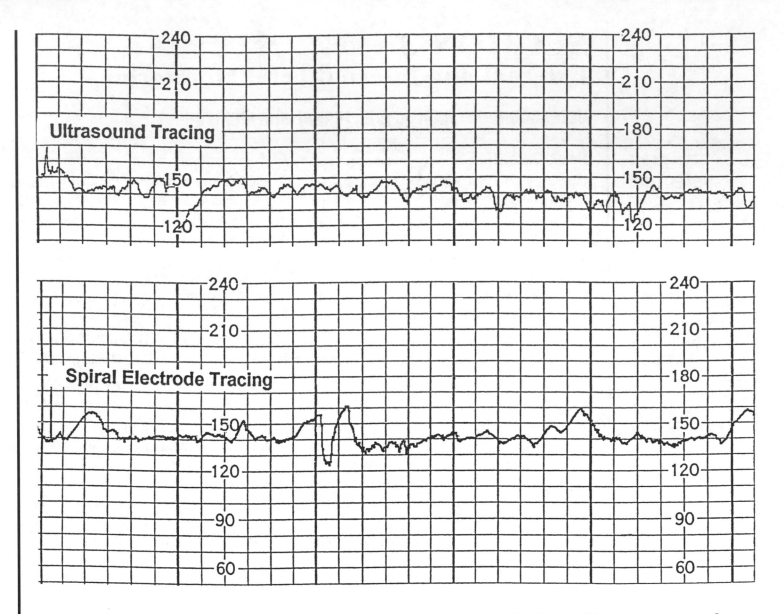

3.1 *With second-generation monitors, the ultrasound tracing is nearly identical in appearance to the spiral electrode tracing. These examples of the fetal heart rate pattern of the same fetus illustrate the similarity before and after spiral electrode use.*

SECOND GENERATION MONITOR SAYINGS

Current sayings about second-generation monitors are:

- *"If it looks GOOD on external, it's probably GOOD on internal."*

- *"If it looks BAD on external, it may be better on internal." "Bad on external" means a smooth tracing which suggests the absence of short-term variability.*

- *"If long-term variability (LTV) and a reactive acceleration are present on external, metabolic acidosis is ruled out and short-term variability (STV) is (conceptually) present."*

ULTRASOUND TRANSDUCER

Ultrasound Transducer (US)

Ultrasound transducers emit high frequency sound waves which cannot be heard by human beings. The ultrasound waveform is interpreted by the computer in the FHR monitor. What you hear **is an artificial sound generated by the monitor**, and you see a rate that is also printed on moving graph paper. When the rates are connected, an FHR pattern appears. It is visually interpreted by the clinician to determine the baseline, accelerations, decelerations, short-term and long-term variability.

COUPLING GEL

Coupling gel (one example is Aquasonic® gel) is applied to the US transducer face to enhance transmission of the US waves. This gel needs to be replaced if the transducer face dries out. Inspect the transducer periodically, especially if gaps occur in the printout. In place of gel, water on gauze can be placed between the transducer face and abdomen.

AUTOMATIC GAIN CONTROL

Automatic gain control is an electronic feature in fetal monitors that strengthens weak signals transmitted by the US or spiral electrode. This feature can strengthen the maternal signal from aortic pulsations, blood flow, or the maternal ECG. In that case, the maternal heart rate (MHR), not the FHR will be printed.

ARTIFACT

Gaps in the FHR printout generated when the US is used occur when there is a weak or inadequately transmitted signal. The gaps and dots are called artifact (see 3.2). Even if a sound is produced by the fetal monitor, do **not** assume that is the FHR. **You must not only hear the sound, but should simultaneously see the FHR printout**. Only then can you be sure that the sound you hear, the rate you see, and the printout accurately reflect the MHR or FHR.

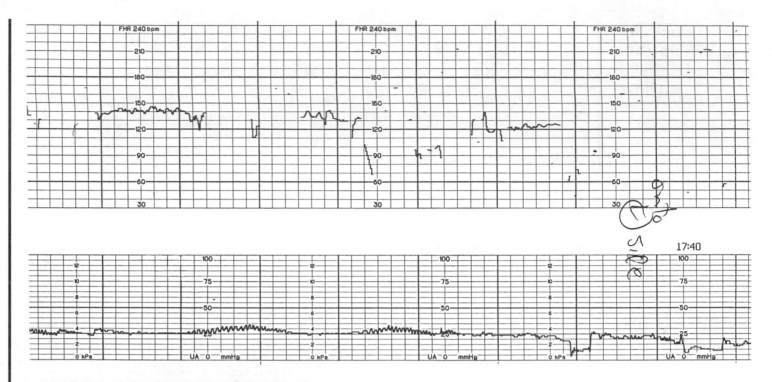

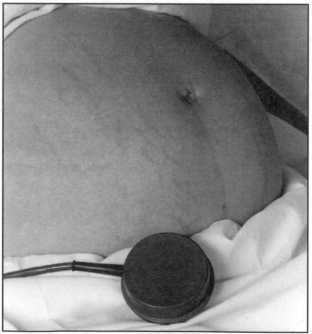

3.2 *Ultrasound tracing with gaps and dots or artifact.*

Testing the US Transducer

To test the US transducer, plug the cable into the monitor, turn the power on, and turn up the sound volume. Apply coupling gel to the transducer face then gently rub the transducer face in small circles, moving in a clockwise direction. Alternatively, hold the face of the dry transducer against your palm while tapping with the fingers of your other hand on the top of the hand holding the transducer. Do you hear static on the fetal monitor? Static means the

3.3 *Ultrasound transducer without coupling gel.*
(Photograph by Pam Barncastle, Castle Studio, Albuquerque, New Mexico).

transducer is working. The absence of static suggests the sensitive crystals in the transducer do not work. If that is the case, that transducer should be sent to the Biomedical Department. It may be unrepairable and will be discarded. Since each fetal monitor component costs hundreds of dollars, handle and store them carefully to prevent damage.

Tocotransducer (TOCO): External Uterine Activity Monitoring

External monitoring of uterine contractions with a tocotransducer reflects uterine activity when the TOCO is placed correctly on the abdomen. The TOCO should be placed above the umbilicus for near term, term, or postterm women, and below the umbilicus for preterm women.

TOCOTRANSDUCER TEST

Testing the Tocotransducer

To test the tocotransducer, plug the cable into its port on the fetal monitor and turn the monitor on. Push the TOCO's pressure-sensitive surface and look at the digital readout on the monitor screen. It may be +199 on Corometrics® monitors or +127 on Hewlett-Packard® monitors. Consult the manufacturer's manual for your monitor. Anything less suggests the TOCO is malfunctioning. When you begin recording, you may reset the TOCO baseline to 10 mm Hg. This is done by pressing the UA ref button or uterine reference button. Review all the buttons on the face of the fetal monitor you will be using. When you use a tocotransducer, the numbers on the fetal monitor paper are insignificant. The exact duration and strength of the contraction cannot be determined. Instead, the uterine activity waveform is examined to determine contraction frequency. Duration is estimated. Palpation is required to determine contraction strength and uterine relaxation between contractions.

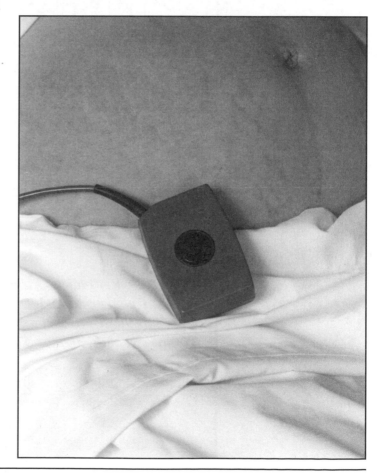

3.4 *The tocotransducer is a pressure-sensitive device that does not require coupling gel. Pressure on the button creates a waveform in the uterine activity channel on the tracing.* (Photograph by Pam Barncastle, Castle Studio, Albuquerque, New Mexico).

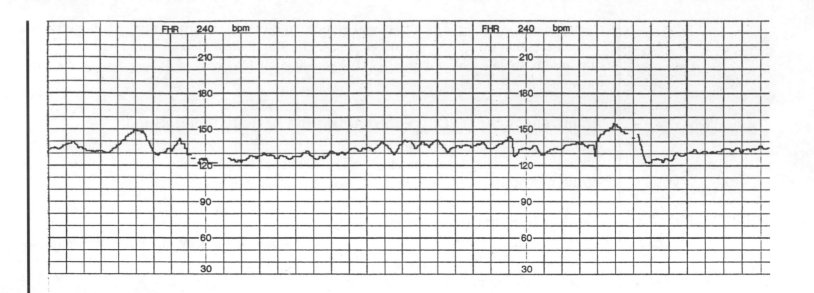

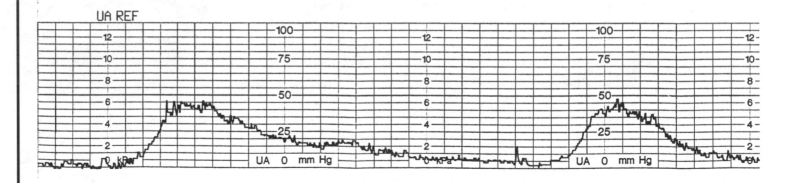

3.5   *UA Ref indicates the fetal monitor automatically adjusted the uterine activity baseline. Contraction frequency and duration are considered relatively accurate when a tocotransducer is used. Duration is 90 to 140 seconds. Palpation of contractions may be done to confirm contraction duration, strength, and relaxation between contractions.*

Internal Monitoring of the Fetal Heart Rate – The Spiral Electrode (SE)

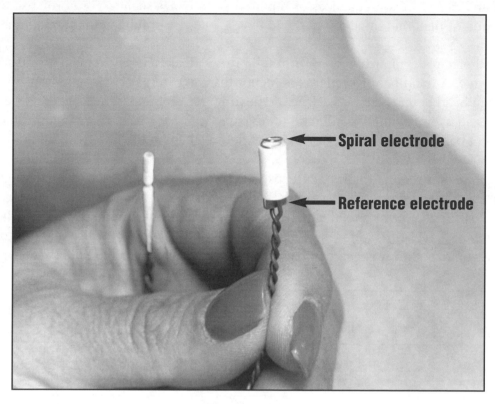

Spiral electrode

Reference electrode

3.6   Spiral electrode. The helix is called a spiral electrode. The metal plate on the opposite side of the plastic tip is called the reference electrode. (Photograph by Pam Barncastle, Castle Studio, Albuquerque, New Mexico).

When ultrasound information is inadequate to make clinical decisions, the application of a spiral electrode to the fetal scalp or buttocks may be needed. The benefit of SE application is that it accurately **measures** the fetal heart rate and short-term variability. The decision to apply an SE is made after weighing risks and benefits. Keep the US transducer on but unplug it. When the spiral electrode is in and working properly, the US may be removed. The SE picks up a direct fetal electrocardiogram signal (FECG) which is transmitted to the fetal monitor along the green or blue wire. On the opposite side of the SE's white plastic tip is a square metal plate or wire. This is the reference electrode. When the reference electrode is in maternal secretions, the maternal electrocardiogram (ECG) is transmitted to the fetal monitor via the red or pink wire. Two ECGs enter the fetal monitor. The green or blue wire transmits the fetal ECG. The red or pink wire transmits the maternal ECG. If the fetus is dead, the maternal ECG will be conducted through the fetus and the green or blue wire, and the maternal heart rate will be printed. That is why it is best to confirm fetal life and the maternal heart rate prior to placement of the spiral electrode or ultrasound transducer. The recorded FHR should be different than the maternal pulse.

A spiral electrode is needed when accelerations are *not* evident and fetal well-being is questioned. Risks of SE application are related to consequences of ruptured membranes such as cord prolapse, infection, scalp abscess, or transmission of maternal infection to the fetus, e.g., herpes or human immunodeficiency virus.

**CONFIRM
FETAL LIFE**

Prior to spiral electrode application, confirm fetal life. Palpate fetal movement or auscultate fetal heart sounds *with a fetoscope*. A hand-held Doppler is no better than an external ultrasound transducer, as both detect motion. When heart sounds are heard, you are hearing the ventricular rate. Other devices, such as a Pinard, a stethoscope, and even an empty cardboard toilet paper roll, have been used to auscultate fetal heart sounds. Of course, a toilet paper roll is not recommended, unless you are in the field without equipment.

DYSRHYTHMIAS

If you auscultate an irregular rhythm, perhaps there is a dysrhythmia such as premature atrial contractions (PACs), premature ventricular contractions (PVCs), or an intermittent second-degree heart block. Since there is a small (< 10%) chance of a fetal cardiac defect, the obstetrician and pediatrician should be notified of an irregular rhythm. A real-time ultrasound may be used to inspect fetal cardiac anatomy and cardiac motion. When an irregular rhythm was heard, the spiral electrode was applied and the FHR pattern looked like this:

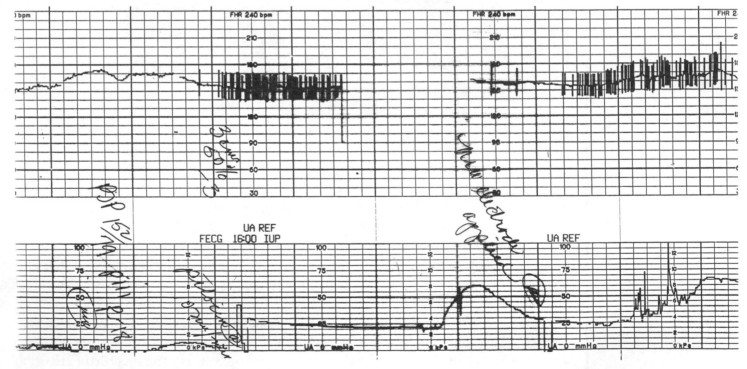

3.7   *Fetal heart rate tracing indicative of premature atrial contractions (lines up and down).*

This irregularity was generated by multiple fetal PACs. **PACs are the most common fetal dysrhythmia**. No treatment or intervention is required. PACs usually resolve after delivery.

ARTIFACT

Artifact appears when the ECG signal transmissions are interrupted. This is especially common with maternal pushing as the electrode wires bounce against the vaginal walls.

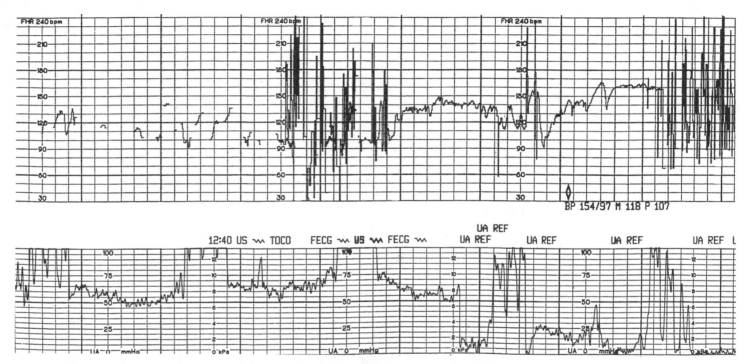

3.8   Dots and gaps represent ultrasound artifact. When a spiral electrode was applied, irregular lines (artifact) indicated the signal transmission was interrupted.

If artifact persists, pull gently on the electrode wires to determine if the electrode fell off. You may need to reapply the ultrasound transducer while a new SE is being inserted or auscultate the FHR to reconfirm fetal life. Also, look under the sheets. The fetus may now be a newborn!

LEG PLATE

All leg plates have a hole into which the end of the spiral electrode is inserted. In 2000, the United States Food and Drug Administration mandated that there be no exposed wires on medical devices (see 3.9).

3.9 ***End of spiral electrode being inserted into leg plate.*** (Photograph by Pam Barncastle, Castle Studio, Albuquerque, New Mexico).

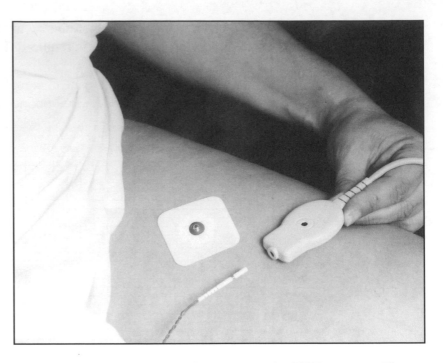

DETERMINING THE FHR

Once the SE is in the fetal tissue, the fetal ECG and maternal ECG can be transmitted to the monitor for analysis. The monitor software identifies the tallest wave in the QRS complexes. The fetal ECG R waves are usually the tallest. The time interval between each set of R waves is determined and a beats per minute (bpm) rate is calculated. For example, if 1/2 second existed between two R waves, the bpm rate would be 120 bpm. A dot is printed at 120 bpm on the fetal heart rate channel. Then, the next R to R interval is determined, and a new bpm rate is printed. Connecting all these dots creates the FHR pattern. If a dysrhythmia occurs, the baseline may not be visible (see 3.10).

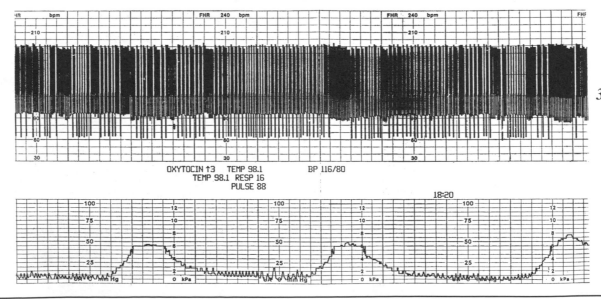

3.10 *A series of fetal multifocal premature ventricular contractions (PVCs) created lines that obscured the baseline.*

You can remove the vertical lines created by PVCs or PACs. There may be a switch or button on the monitor that can be activated to delete these lines. Hewlett-Packard® calls this "logic." Corometrics® calls it the "ECG artifact elimination" switch. Find this switch or button on the fetal monitor.

3.11 Spacelabs® monitors have an ECG plot feature.

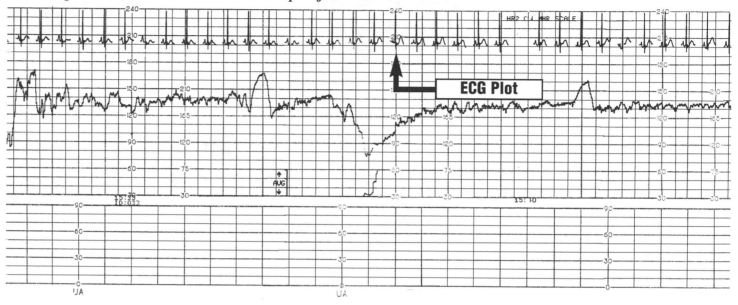

ECG PLOT

Some machines have no logic button, but instead can print the fetal ECG for waveform analysis, e.g., Spacelabs® monitors and Oxford Medical's Sonicaid® intrapartum monitor. The ECG plot can be turned on or off in the Spacelabs® monitor (see 3.12). A button is depressed to plot the FECG on Sonicaid® fetal monitor paper.

Review your equipment with a skilled clinician. Identify:

- the spiral electrode
- the reference electrode
- the leg plate
- the "logic" button or ECG plot switch.

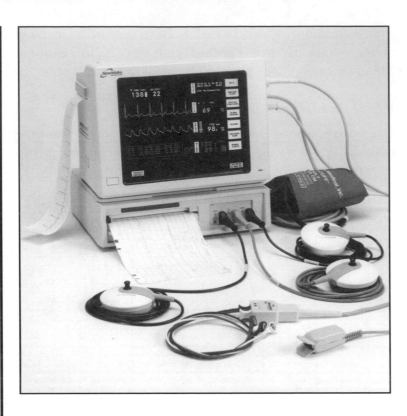

3.12 *Spacelabs® monitor with capability of monitoring maternal blood pressure, oxygen saturation, pulse, and temperature. It also has an ECG printer, maternal pulse oximeter, maternal ECG cable, tocotransducer and two ultrasound transducers.* (Photograph courtesy of Spacelabs Medical, Redmond, Washington.)

Internal Monitoring of Uterine Contractions with an Intrauterine Pressure Catheter (IUPC)

PREPARING TO INSERT THE IUPC

When accurate information is needed regarding uterine contraction frequency, duration, strength, and resting tone, or an amnioinfusion is needed, an intrauterine pressure catheter (IUPC) is inserted.

Prior to IUPC insertion, gather the following items:
1. IUPC

2. IUPC cable (also called the IUPC/monitor interface cable)

3. Sterile gloves.

Carefully open the IUPC package maintaining aseptic technique. If you are using a transducer-tipped catheter, attach the IUPC to the interface cable and plug the cable into the fetal monitor. The IUPC-cable-fetal monitor system can now be "zeroed" prior to insertion. Ask a skilled clinician to demonstrate how this is done. Transducer-tipped IUPC systems never need to be rezeroed unless part of the system changes, for example, if you change the fetal monitor, you'll need to rezero the system.

The membranes must be ruptured prior to IUPC insertion. If an artificial rupture of membranes (AROM) is done, record the time of the AROM and the color, amount, and odor of the amniotic fluid. Also record the fetal heart rate prior to and after the AROM. Once the IUPC is inserted, it is recommended that you establish and document the baseline pressure readings with her on her right side, left side, and semi-Fowler's.

If an amnioinfusion is ordered, normal saline or lactated Ringer's solution is infused. Usually a 200 to 500 milliliters or more bolus is infused at room temperature followed by 60 to 180 milliliters per hour. An infusion warmer or blood warmer is used for amnioinfusion of preterm gestations. Monitor the FHR closely. If it worsens after the amnioinfusion is started, stop the infusion and notify the midwife or physician. Inspect the linen protector regularly to confirm fluid is leaving the uterus. Every 2 hours after rupture of membranes, assess the maternal temperature and pulse and note any foul smelling amniotic fluid or uterine tenderness. Record the color, amount, and odor of the fluid. A rising temperature or rising maternal or fetal heart rate should be reported as they are associated with chorioamnionitis. Since amnioinfusion increases the amount of liquid in the uterus, you may see a rise in the recorded resting tone and contraction peak pressure as both recordings also reflect hydrostatic pressure.

INTRAUTERINE PRESSURES

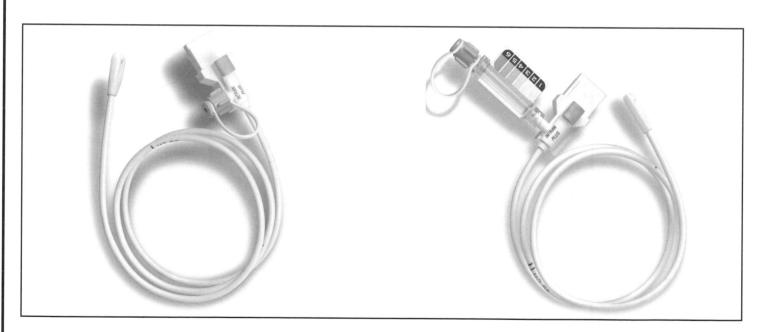

3.13   Intran™ Plus intrauterine pressure catheters with and without a color strip for meconium-stained amniotic fluid color comparisons. (Photograph courtesy of Utah Medical Products Inc., Midvale, Utah.)

The four components of pressure that may be transmitted by the IUPC to the fetal monitor are:

- hydrostatic pressure
- elastic recoil of the uterine wall (uterine tonus)
- contraction pressure
- atmospheric pressure.

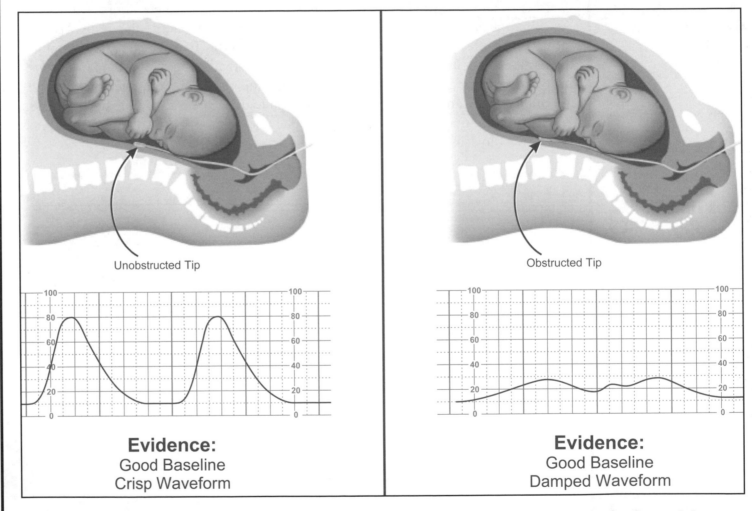

Unobstructed Tip	Obstructed Tip
Evidence: Good Baseline Crisp Waveform	**Evidence:** Good Baseline Damped Waveform

3.14 *Even when the IUPC is properly inserted in the amniotic sac, the waveform may be damped due to an obstruction.*

For accurate measurement, it is vital that the IUPC be placed within the amniotic space. Transducer-tipped IUPCs are less susceptible to an obstruction due to their recessed pressure port. But if a damped waveform is suspected, rotation of the transducer-tipped IUPC may help improve the tracing. It may be helpful to flush liquid-filled IUPCs to remove debris from the multiple ports at the end of the IUPC and to eliminate air bubbles that might have formed if the IUPC tip were in a dry pocket.

It is important to verify IUPC placement by asking the woman to cough. There should be a sharp spike on the IUPC tracing when she coughs. If after insertion of the IUPC tip past the fetal head resistance persists, a rare possibility is that the IUPC is outside of the sac, between the chorion and uterine wall. This extraovular insertion may cause bleeding as well as a damped waveform. Notify the midwife or physician.

ZEROING THE SYSTEM

Zeroing the System

Learn about the IUPC used at your hospital. If you use a liquid-filled IUPC, flush the catheter prior to insertion. Be sure to use sterile water or sterile saline without a preservative, because preservatives, such as benzyl alcohol, have been linked to intraventricular bleeding in preterm fetuses. Then zero the IUPC-cable-monitor system. Zeroing is the process of electronically removing atmospheric pressure from the tracing so that the recorded uterine activity waveform will only include

- hydrostatic pressure

- elastic recoil of the uterus (uterine tonus) and

- contraction pressure.

It is best to zero the IUPC-cable-monitor system prior to insertion. Some IUPC systems never need to be rezeroed. For example, if the Intran® IUPC system is zeroed prior to insertion, it should not need to be rezeroed unless a part of the IUPC-cable-fetal monitor system is changed. Consult the manufacturer's guidelines.

CABLE OFFSET

"Cable offset" is an electronic feature that adds or subtracts 2 mm Hg from the total uterine pressure reading due to cable and pressure transducer design. This"offset" will be removed if the IUPC-cable-monitor system is zeroed **prior** to insertion.

HYDROSTATIC PRESSURE

Hydrostatic Pressure

The pressure exerted by the weight of the amniotic fluid above the IUPC pressure sensitive transducer is called hydrostatic pressure. Hydrostatic pressure varies depending on the location of the IUPC pressure sensitive transducer in relation to the amniotic fluid above it. The transducer may be in the IUPC tip or located outside the uterus in the cable or as a separate device attached to the IUPC with its own cable to the fetal monitor. No matter where it is, **hydrostatic pressure will always be a part of the recorded pressures**. Hydrostatic pressure changes 5 to 10 mm Hg when the maternal position changes. Hydrostatic pressure increases when the pressure sensitive transducer is below a column of amniotic fluid and decreases when the transducer is near the top or above the column of amniotic fluid. Amnioinfusion can increase hydrostatic pressure.

ELASTIC RECOIL/RESTING TONE

Elastic Recoil/Resting Tone

Elastic recoil is the normal tension or uterine tonus exerted by tissues in and around the uterus. Hydrostatic pressure plus uterine tonus produce the resting tone recorded between contractions. The time between contractions is called the interval. The normal resting tone range is 5 to 25 mm Hg. Determine the resting tone after IUPC insertion with the woman on her left side, right side, and semi-Fowler's so that you have 3 baselines should you later chose to add fluid with an amnioinfusion. The added fluid can increase hydrostatic pressure and change the resting tone. Are you sure fluid is leaving the uterus?

PEAK IUP

Peak IUP

The top of the uterine activity waveform when an IUPC is in the uterus is called the peak intrauterine pressure or peak IUP. Peak pressures tend to diminish when the uterus ruptures. In that case, there may still be palpable contractions, but the IUPC will often be outside of the uterus and absolutely no waveform will be recorded. The most accurate recording of uterine activity including the frequency, duration, resting tone, interval, and peak IUP is obtained when the IUPC is transducer-tipped. All other IUPC systems have the pressure-sensing transducer outside of the uterus which introduces varying degrees of error in signal transmission to the fetal monitor.

IUPC RISKS

IUPC Risks

Risks associated with IUPC use include:
- infection

- uterine perforation

- umbilical cord injury or entanglement

- placental injury such as abruption and

- extraovular placement.

If after IUPC insertion there is a soft, nontender, contracting uterus, but no uterine recorded waveform, suspect uterine perforation. Sometimes perforation is asymptomatic. If, after insertion, there is vaginal bleeding and uterine hyperstimulation, suspect a placental abruption.

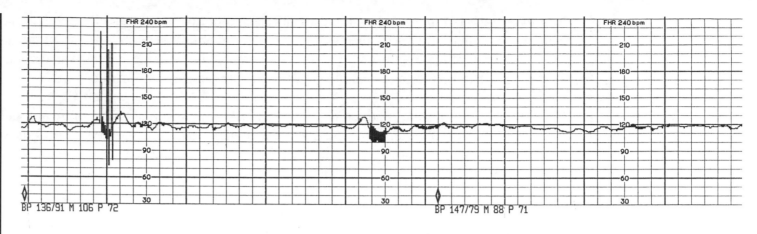

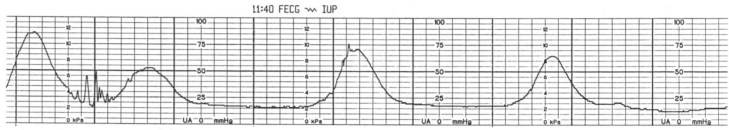

3.15 *An intrauterine pressure catheter was used to record contractions with a peak pressure of approximately 53 to 85 mm Hg and a resting tone of 13 to 18 mm Hg.*

SUMMARY

Summary
Autocorrelation has changed fetal monitoring by improving analysis of the ultrasound signal. The printed rate is within 2.5 bpm of the true rate. If the fetal heart rate tracing looks good when the US (external monitor) is used, it will probably look good when the spiral electrode (internal monitor) is used. Therefore, application of internal devices should be considered only after the risks and benefits have been weighed.

Testing of the tocotransducer and ultrasound transducer, and proper placement are critical to the recording of accurate, interpretable data. Confirm fetal life. Palpate fetal movement or auscultate with a fetoscope, especially if a dysrhythmia is suspected. Determine fetal position and the gestational age prior to transducer application.

The spiral electrode is used to transmit a direct fetal electrocardiogram (FECG) signal into the fetal monitor. When the fetus is dead, the maternal ECG will be conducted through the fetal body into the spiral electrode and cable. Use of the spiral electrode should be conveyed to the newborn nurse so that the puncture site may be observed during hospitalization.

Prior to use, the intrauterine pressure catheter-cable-monitor system should be zeroed according to the manufacturer's guidelines to remove the electronic offset and atmospheric pressure from the uterine activity tracing. The tracing will reflect hydrostatic pressure in combination with uterine tonus and contractions. The maximum normal resting tone (uterine tonus plus hydrostatic pressure) is 25 mm Hg.

Since membranes must be ruptured to insert the IUPC, the maternal temperature and pulse should be taken every 2 hours. The color, amount, and odor of the amniotic fluid, e.g., nonfoul or foul, should be assessed and recorded when the linen protector is changed. The midwife and/or physician should be notified of any bleeding, abnormal fetal heart rate pattern, a damped IUPC waveform, abnormal vital signs, foul smelling amniotic fluid, and uterine tenderness. The amnioinfusion should be discontinued until the woman has been evaluated.

EXERCISES

Exercises

Examine these four tracings. Fill in the blanks under each one.

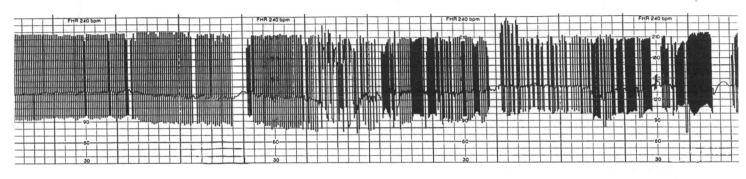

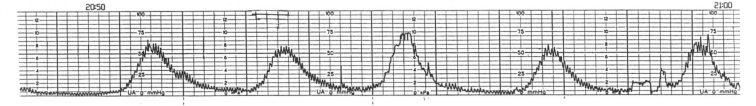

3.16   Recurrent fetal PACs. Tocotransducer is in place. Apgar scores were 5 and 9 at 1 and 5 minutes.

1.   Contraction frequency = _____ minutes

2.   Contraction duration = _____ seconds

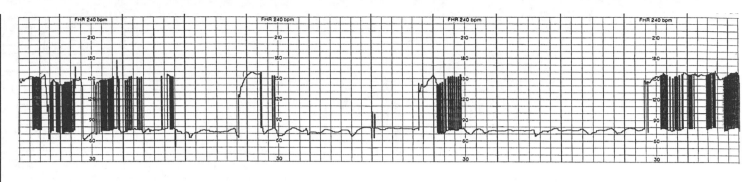

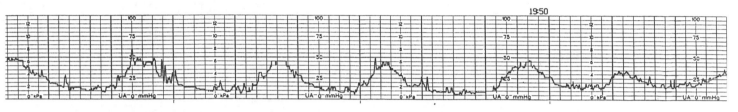

3.17 *Dropped beats and bradycardia reflecting a Mobitz II second-degree heart block. Tocotransducer is in place. Apgar scores were 5 and 9 at 1 and 5 minutes.*

3.   Contraction frequency = _____ minutes

4.   Contraction duration = _____ seconds

3.18 *Unifocal PVCs. Tocotransducer is in place. Apgar scores were 8 and 9 at 1 and 5 minutes.*

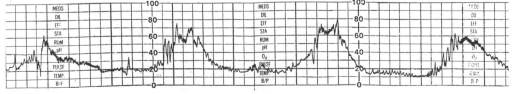

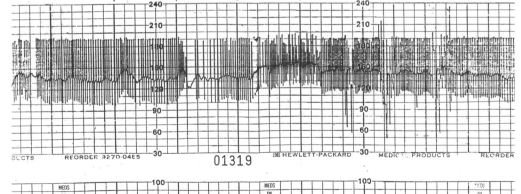

5. Contraction frequency = _____ minutes

6. Contraction duration = _____ seconds

7. Contraction peak IUP = _____ mm Hg

8. Contraction resting tone = _____ mm Hg

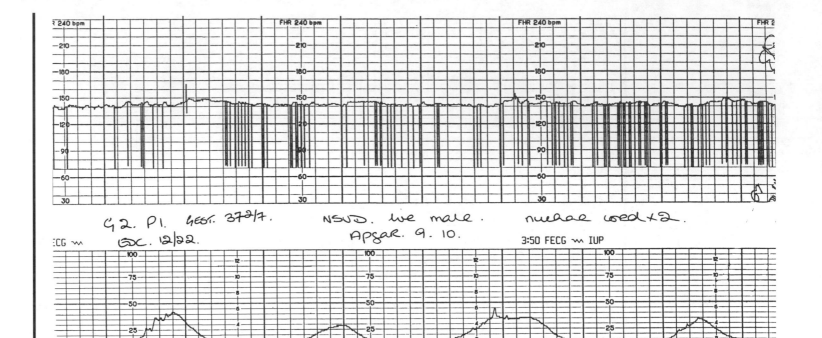

G2. P1. GEST. 37 2/7. NSVD. we male. nuchal cord x2.
EDC. 12/22. Apgar. 9. 10.
ECG ~ 3:50 FECG ~ IUP

3.19   Dropped beats due to a Mobitz II second-degree heart block.

    9.   Contraction frequency = _____ minutes

   10.   Contraction duration = _____ seconds

   11.   Contraction peak IUP = _____ mm Hg

   12.   Contraction resting tone = _____ mm Hg

Answers on page 51.

1. every 2 minutes
2. 70-90 seconds
3. every 2 minutes
4. 60-70 seconds
5. every 2-2$^1/2$ minutes

6. 80 seconds
7. cannot determine with a tocotransducer in place
8. cannot determine with a tocotransducer in place

9. every 2-2$^1/2$ minutes
10. 50-90 seconds
11. 30-40 mm Hg
12. 12-15 mm Hg

SECTION 3: EXTERNAL AND INTERNAL FETAL MONITORING

QUESTIONS

QUESTIONS

Directions: Circle T if the statement is true, F if it is false.

T   F   1. Always keep the ultrasound transducer on the abdomen until the spiral electrode is in and working.

T   F   2. Coupling gel helps transmit fetal heart sounds when it is applied to the ultrasound transducer.

T   F   3. When "logic" is on it removes abnormal fetal heart rate lines due to premature atrial contractions and premature ventricular contractions.

T   F   4. Zeroing removes the effect of hydrostatic pressure on the uterine activity printout.

T   F   5. Offset is ± 2 mm Hg in the uterine pressure due to the cable and pressure transducer design.

T   F   6. Autocorrelation creates a more reliable external tracing than first-generation peak detection.

T   F   7. A spiral electrode and/or ultrasound transducer can transmit the maternal heart rate.

T   F   8. The ultrasound transducer transmits the electrical energy of the heartbeat.

T   F   9. Confirmation of fetal life can best be accomplished by using a hand-held doppler if the ultrasound transducer failed to detect the fetal heart rate.

T   F   10. Maternal tachycardia occurs when there is chorioamnionitis.

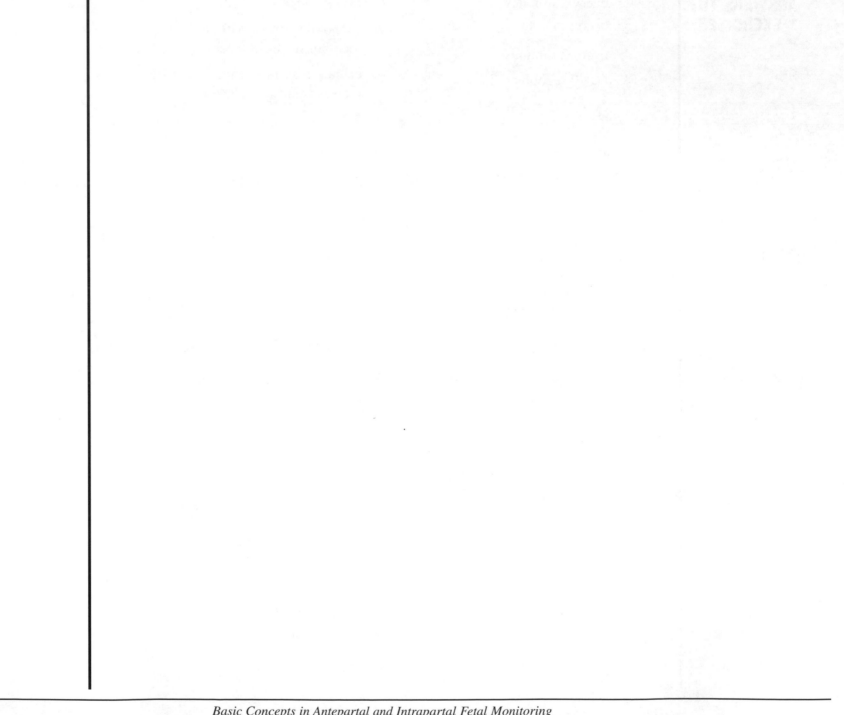

SECTION 4
Uterine Contractions

UTERINE PHYSIOLOGY

Uterine Physiology

The uterus is controlled by involuntary muscle fibers. Alpha receptors in the uterine muscle cells stimulate uterine contractions, and beta receptors stimulate uterine relaxation. Norepinephrine and epinephrine stimulate both alpha and beta receptors. Prior to labor, estrogen stimulates the alpha receptors, and progesterone stimulates the beta receptors. During pregnancy, progesterone and estrogen levels are balanced. Progesterone levels drop, and estrogen exerts a dominant influence on the uterus prior to the onset of labor. The increase of estrogen and decrease of progesterone stimulates the formation of oxytocin receptors in the uterine muscle cells. The uterine cells begin to communicate by spreading their energy (action potential) through portals called gap junctions. This leads to synchronous uterine muscle cell contractions. Cocaine and thrombin can also stimulate contraction of uterine muscle cells.

PACEMAKERS

It is theorized that specialized cells in the fundus of the uterus initiate an electrical impluse that stimulates a contraction. These cells are called pacemakers.

IMPULSE PATH

A normal contraction begins in the fundus and proceeds symmetrically downward toward the cervix. Asymmetry results when the uterine cells function independently causing ineffective uterine contractions and minimal dilatation. Ketones in the urine during labor are often associated with ineffective uterine contractions. Therefore, it is important to provide adequate caloric intake either through hydration therapy, e.g., a controlled intravenous infusion of a dextrose-containing solution at 125 ml/hour, or by ingestion of glucose-containing liquids.

FEAR RESULTS IN INEFFECTIVE CONTRACTIONS

Fear causes the release of catecholamines (epinephrine and norepinephrine) which have an effect on uterine activity. Norepinephrine binds with alpha receptors to increase uterine resting tone, contraction frequency, duration, and strength. Epinephrine, secreted in small amounts, binds with beta receptors and decreases uterine activity. The overall uterine response to maternal fear is more frequent but **ineffective** contractions that can even arrest labor progress. This is why many women, who think they are in labor, contract so much more when they first arrive at the hospital than they do after they calm down. When a woman's anxiety decreases, contractions become more effective though less frequent.

FEAR ⇒ CATECHOLAMINES ⇒ INCREASED BUT INEFFECTIVE UTERINE ACTIVITY

The woman's childbirth preparation, coping skills, and support system affect her response to contractions. A doula can help the woman minimize the effect of fear on her uterine activity and shorten the duration of labor.

Contraction Concepts

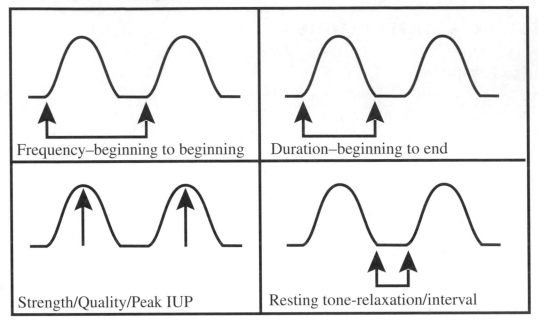

Frequency–beginning to beginning

Duration–beginning to end

Strength/Quality/Peak IUP

Resting tone-relaxation/interval

4.1   Contraction concepts

PALPATION

A contraction occurs when the uterine muscle cells shorten. The uterus becomes more globular and tilts forward. You can feel this when your hand is on the fundus and your other hand is on the lower abdomen.

Palpation of resting tone is an important element in ongoing assessment. Ideally, contractions should be 60 or more seconds apart. This resting period, or interval, allows optimal delivery of oxygen to the fetus and removal of carbon dioxide from the fetus.

DEFINITION OF TERMS

FREQUENCY

Contraction frequency is calculated in minutes from the beginning of one contraction to the beginning of the next contraction. It can be charted as "UCs q 4," meaning uterine contractions every 4 minutes.

DURATION

Contraction duration is timed from the beginning to the end of a contraction. It can be charted as UCs x 30-40 meaning contractions last 30-40 seconds.

INTERVAL

The **interval** is the time from the end of one contraction to the beginning of the next contraction. It should last 60 or more seconds so that fetal oxygen can be replenished. Resting tone is assessed during the interval. Interval duration is not documented.

HYPER-STIMULATION

When the interval is less than 1 minute, and the frequency is closer than every 2 minutes, uterine hyperstimulation exists. Hyperstimulation may occur with an abruption or cocaine, oxytocin, or prostaglandin use.

PEAK IUP

Peak intrauterine pressure (IUP) is usually higher than 35 mm Hg and may exceed 100 mm Hg during pushing. The peak is charted as "UCs ⇑ 80-90," meaning peak IUP ranges between 80 and 90 mm Hg.

INTENSITY

Intensity is measured as the difference between peak IUP and resting tone. Another name for intensity is **active pressure**. Montevideo units (discussed below) are calculated by adding intensity of each contraction in a 10 minute period. Contraction intensity can **only** be measured with an IUPC in place.

STRENGTH/ QUALITY

Strength or quality of contractions is judged at the contraction's peak. Push gently on the abdomen near the top of the uterus. Classify the contraction strength as mild, moderate or strong.

Mild   ⇒   abdomen easily indents to feel uterus, feels like pressing on your cheek

Moderate ⇒   abdomen firmer, some indentation occurs, feels like pressing on your nose

Strong   ⇒   abdomen feels hard and cannot be indented, feels like pressing on your forehead

Strength with an intrauterine pressure catheter (IUPC) is the peak IUP on the uterine activity waveform. Documentation should include frequency, duration, peak IUP or strength, and relaxation or resting tone. For example, "UCs q 4-5 x 30-40, ⇑ 50-60, with resting tone 10-15."

RESTING TONE

Resting tone is the pressure exerted by uterine muscle cells and supportive tissues when they are at rest. The IUPC printout of resting tone always includes hydrostatic pressure. Resting tone between contractions should be 5 to 25 mm Hg, but is often closer to 8 to 12 mm Hg or soft to palpation.

HYPERTONUS

A resting tone greater than 25 mm Hg is called **hypertonus**. Resting tone may be documented as "rest tone 30-35" meaning 30-35 mm Hg (when an intrauterine pressure catheter is in place) or "firm between contractions" when resting tone is palpated. This is abnormal.

MONTEVIDEO UNITS

Montevideo Units (MVUs)
The original formula by Drs. Caldeyro-Barcia and Alvarez in 1952 was
   MVUs = the *sum* of each contraction's *peak minus* the *resting tone* in a 10 minute period.

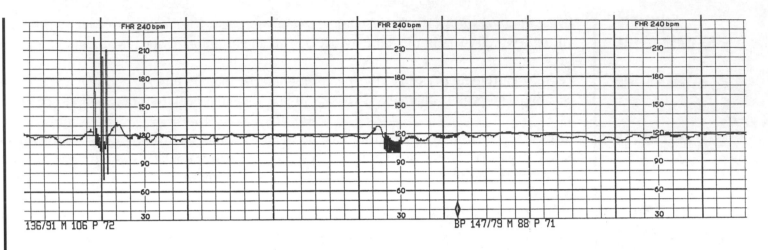

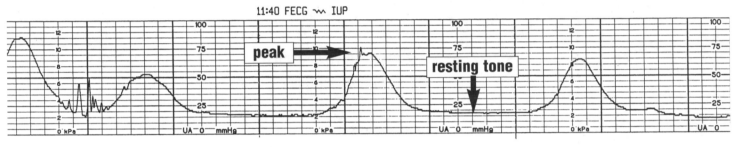

4.2 *MVUs are calculated by adding the active pressure or intensity in 10 minutes. Intensity is the contraction peak minus resting tone.*

There are 4 contractions with peak pressures of approximately 85, 55, 70, and 65 mm Hg. Resting tone averages 15 mm Hg. 85-15 + 55-15 + 70-15 + 65-15 = 70 + 40 + 55 + 50 or 215 Montevideo Units or MVUs.

ADEQUATE LABOR PROGRESS

Drs. Caldeyro-Barcia and Alvarez found that 150 to 250 MVUs were associated with adequate labor progress. Normal labors have ranged from 66 to 340 MVUs with an average of 100 in early labor, 200 by 10 cm dilatation, and 250 while pushing. MVUs are higher during ambulation (73 to 205) versus lying supine (80 to 176). Hypocontractile labors have lower MVUs (21 to 313), yet can overlap values for normal labors. Therefore, MVUs should *not* be used to identify hypocontractility.

Maximize MVUs and labor progress by having the woman assume an upright position, and act to decrease maternal anxiety and increase maternal comfort.

Assessment of the maternal response to labor and palpation of contractions is more important in managing labor than calculation of MVUs. Often MVUs are calculated when Pitocin® is infusing. MVUs between 150 and 250 suggest that dilatation and fetal descent should be occurring.

A third way to calculate MVUs is to add the mm Hg as you move from the base of each contraction to its peak. Adding all contractions in 10 minutes gives you the MVUs.

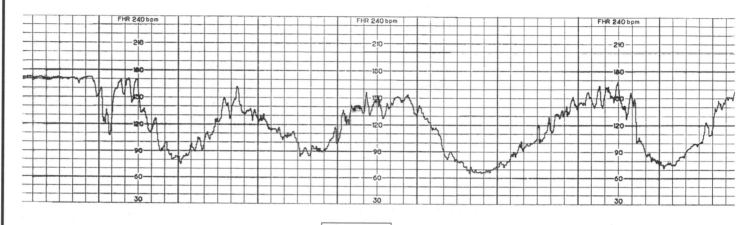

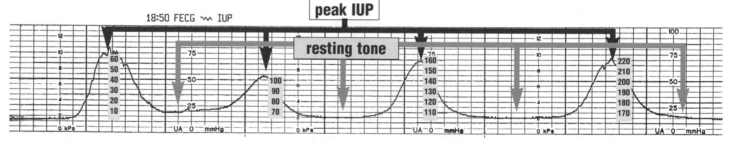

4.3   *Calculate MVUs by adding the mm Hg under each contraction over a ten minute period. In this example there are 220 MVUs. 10 mm Hg was used as the resting tone.*

EXERCISES

Exercises
Calculate the Montevideo Units

1.   Peak pressures   50, 60, 70, 60 mm Hg
      Resting tone   10   mm Hg
      MVUs   _____

2.   Peak pressures   50, 65   mm Hg
        Resting tone   5   mm Hg
        MVUs   _____

3.   Peak pressures   100, 85, 75   mm Hg
        Resting tone   25   mm Hg
        MVUs   _____

See the answers on page 71.

Another way to calculate MVUs is to calculate the average peak IUP in 10 minutes, subtract the average resting tone, and multiply that number by the number of contractions. For example, if the peak pressures are 60, 75, and 90 mm Hg, their average peak is 60 + 75 + 90 ÷ 3 or 75. If the average resting tone is 15 mm Hg, 75 minus 15 is 60 mm Hg, 60 times 3 contractions in 10 minutes is 180 MVUs. With 180 MVUs you would expect adequate labor progress.

NORMAL LABOR CONTRACTION FEATURES

Normal Labor Contraction Features

- fundal dominance
- coordinated/symmetrical movement
- 2 - 5 contractions each 10 minutes
- 45 - 90 seconds duration
- 40 - 60 mm Hg peak IUP early first stage
- 70 - ≥100 mm Hg peak IUP late first stage and second stage.

DYSTOCIA FEATURES

Abnormal Labor (Dystocia) Features

- no fundal dominance (discoordinate contractions)
- no cervical change or abnormally slow cervical change
- mixed "subnormal" and normal patterns that are ineffective for dilatation and effacement
- presenting part is not well applied to the cervix
- usually responds well to oxytocin augmentation, hydration, and/or narcotics.

The frequency, duration, and or peak/strength of contractions may help identify abnormal uterine activity. You can also plot a labor curve to graphically assess labor progress.

LABOR CURVE

The purpose of plotting a labor curve is to visualize the progress of dilatation and descent. Graph paper is used to plot these values. The hospital's chart form may have a space for you to plot a labor curve.

4.4 **A sequence of observations of cervical dilatation and fetal station is entered on graph paper to display labor progress with the passage of time.** (Cohen, W. R. and Friedman, E. A. (1983). Management of Labor. University Park Press.)

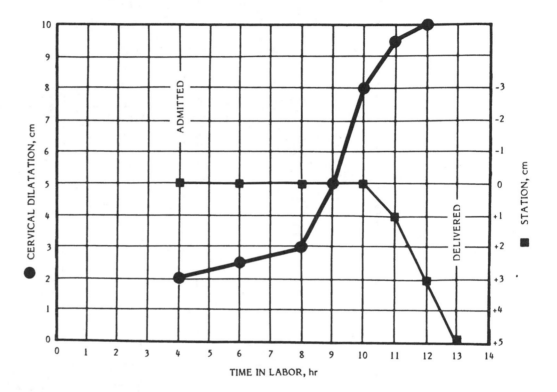

If, after 2 or more hours of active labor, there is no progress in dilatation, an arrest of labor may exist. The woman should be evaluated by the midwife or physician. In addition, the midwife and/or physician should be called if:

- there is a failure to dilate, perhaps the fetus is not well applied to the cervix or the contractions are weak and ineffective.

- after 10 cm dilatation there is no descent after 1 or more hours of pushing. This is called an arrest of descent.

- after some initial descent there is an arrest of descent, pushing efforts may be weak. An upright position might help. If the fetal or pelvic size limit descent, a cesarean section may be needed.

Benefits of Using the Tocotransducer (TOCO)

- provides a record of the contraction pattern and its relationship to the FHR

- noninvasive

- provides information about uterine contraction frequency, duration, and waveform configuration

- may be a closer representation of the *onset and duration* of contractions than reported by the woman or her coach

- suggests fetal movement (spikes) and/or maternal breathing (rhythmic up and down fluctuations).

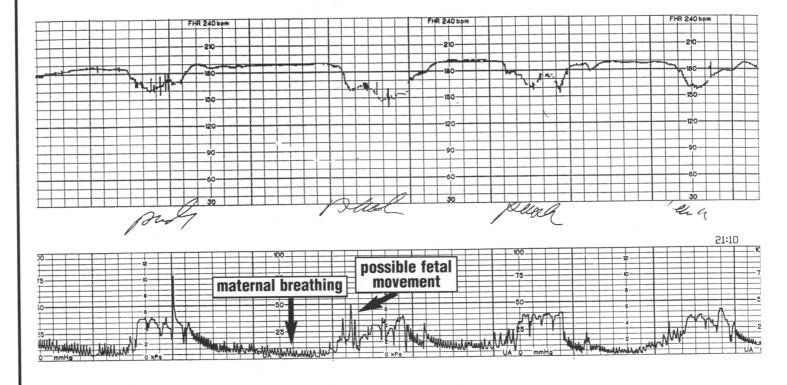

4.5 *Pushing creates a picket fence appearance. Between and during contractions, spikes suggest fetal movement. Fetal movement should be confirmed by palpation. The up and down small fluctuations between contractions suggest maternal breathing at a rate of approximately 28/minute. Hyperventilation may decrease oxygen delivery to the fetus. Coach the woman to slow down her breathing.*

Tocotransducer Limitations

- the TOCO should be placed above the woman's umbilicus in near-term to postterm pregnancies and at or below the umbilicus in preterm gestations

- incorrect positioning of the TOCO may lead to the incorrect detection of the contractions

- contractions in preterm pregnancies may be difficult to record because the electronic fetal monitor TOCO is not as sensitive as a home uterine monitor created specifically for preterm gestations

- subcutaneous tissue, especially in obese women, can interfere with the detection of contractions.

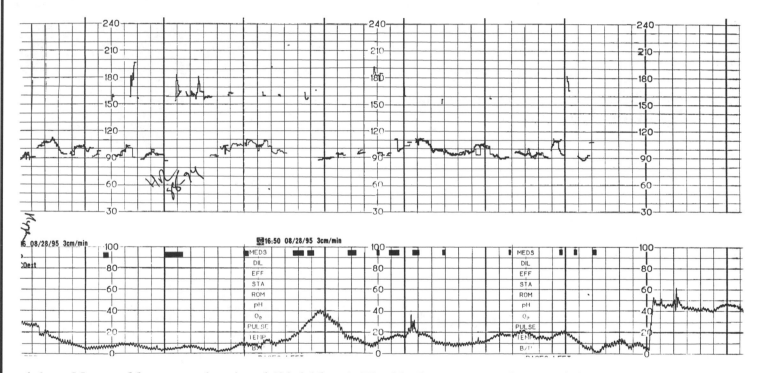

4.6   Maternal heart rate is printed (88-94 bpm). The black squares at the top of the uterine activity channel may reflect maternal aortic movement or artifact because they occur when no clear fetal heart rate is printed. The FHR or doubling of the maternal heart rate is intermittently recorded near 160 bpm. Contractions may or may not be too close together. Both the ultrasound transducer and TOCO need to be adjusted before making clinical decisions related to the fetal status and uterine activity.

IUPC INDICATIONS

Indications for Intrauterine Pressure Monitoring (IUPC)

The use of an IUPC is based on a cost/benefit analysis. Risks of IUPC insertion include placental abruption, entanglement with the umbilical cord, lower segment uterine perforation, infection, and extraovular placement. IUPCs may be used:

- to evaluate contractions during abnormal (as well as normal) labor
- to evaluate uterine activity during a TOLAC (Trial of Labor After Cesarean) or in women with a history of uterine surgery
- to accurately monitor contractions during augmentation or induction
- to more closely examine and interpret the relationship between contractions and FHR decelerations, and
- to evaluate the actual contraction frequency, duration, peak IUP, and resting tone.

UTERINE ACTIVITY VARIATIONS

Variations in Uterine Activity

The uterine activity pattern may vary. Examples of variations include

- coupling
- hyperstimulation
- hypertonus
- uterine reversal
- tetanic contractions, and
- low amplitude high frequency (LAHF) waves or uterine irritability.

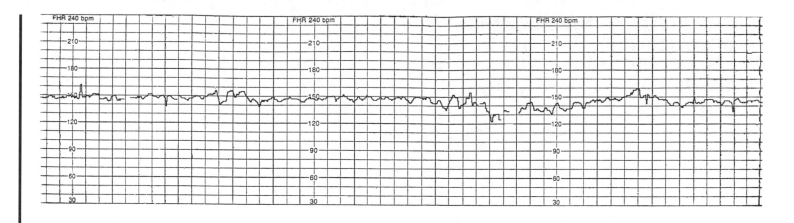

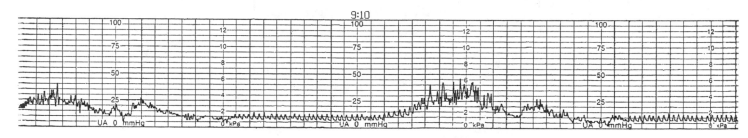

4.7   During coupling, the first contraction is always longer than the second.

Coupling

Coupling is often seen when the fetus is in an occiput posterior (looking up) position or OT (occiput transverse) position (looking sideways). To document coupling in this example, you might chart "UCs q 5 x 40-80, mild - mod with coupling." Of course, strength will be palpated. Or you could document "coupling q 5 x 40-80, mild - mod." The latter example is easier to visualize in your mind.

Hyperstimulation

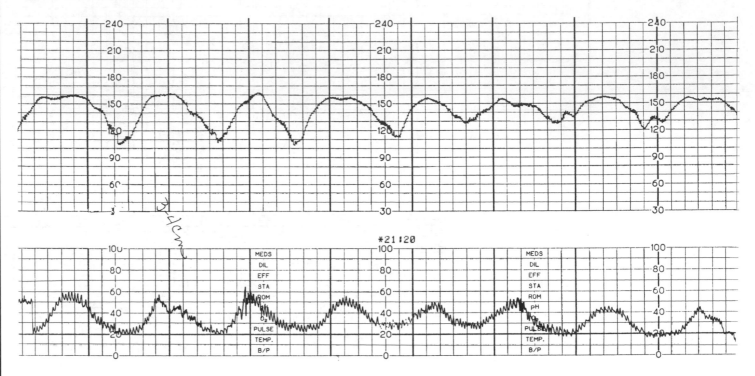

4.8 *The frequency of contractions is approximately every minute with an interval of only a few seconds between contractions. There are late decelerations with a FHR baseline level of 155-160 bpm. This is a classic abruption pattern and a medical emergency. When the fetus demonstrates an abnormal heart rate with uterine hyperstimulation, it is called hyperstimulation syndrome.*

Hyperstimulation is often associated with Pitocin® or prostaglandin sensitivity or abruption. Pitocin® or prostaglandins should be discontinued or removed if hyperstimulation occurs. Restart Pitocin® at half of the dose once hyperstimulation ceases and an abruption is ruled out. Also, determine if the woman has used cocaine or smokes cigarettes, as both increase the risk of abruption.

Hypertonus

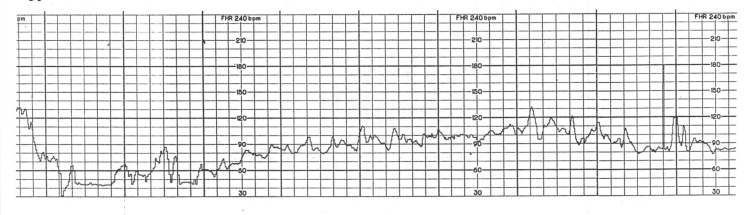

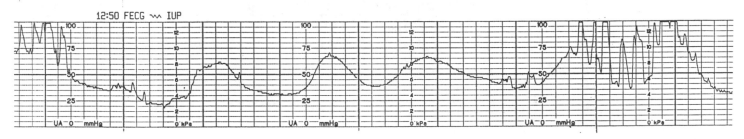

4.9 Uterine hypertonus often accompanies hyperstimulation. Hypertonus is a resting tone above 25 mm Hg.

In this example, the first and last contraction indicate maternal pushing. There is hyperstimulation and hypertonus. The fetus is bradycardic. If Pitocin® is infusing, it should be stopped immediately. The woman should be positioned on her side and encouraged to stop pushing. An intravenous bolus of 500 ml lactated Ringer's solution may decrease uterine activity. Oxygen should be administered at 8 or more liters per minute (LPM) by a simple face mask or 12 LPM by a partial rebreathing mask. A vaginal examination should be done to rule out umbilical cord prolapse and to assess dilatation, effacement and station. If delivery is imminent, an upright position is best to expedite delivery. The midwife or physician should be promptly notified.

Uterine Reversal

If the TOCO is placed low on the abdomen or over the baby's buttocks and the fetus pulls away during the contraction, a negative instead of positive pressure will be exerted. This creates a reversed image or uterine reversal pattern. If the woman is asleep, there is no need to adjust the TOCO as the tracing provides adequate information for decision making (see 4.10).

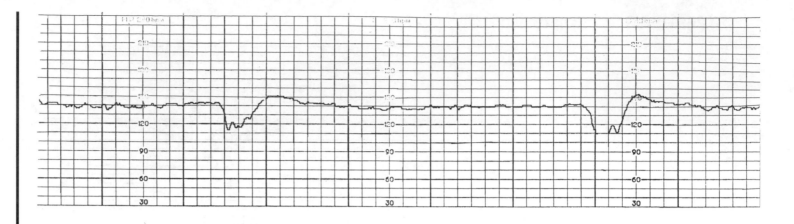

US ∿ TOCO 3 CM/MIN

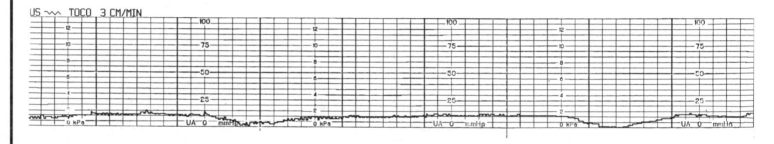

4.10   *The FHR reflects variable decelerations with overshoots. The baseline is 136-142 bpm with minimal long-term variability. Contractions are reversed with a frequency of every 4¹/₂ minutes and a duration of approximately 70 seconds.*

Tetanic Contractions

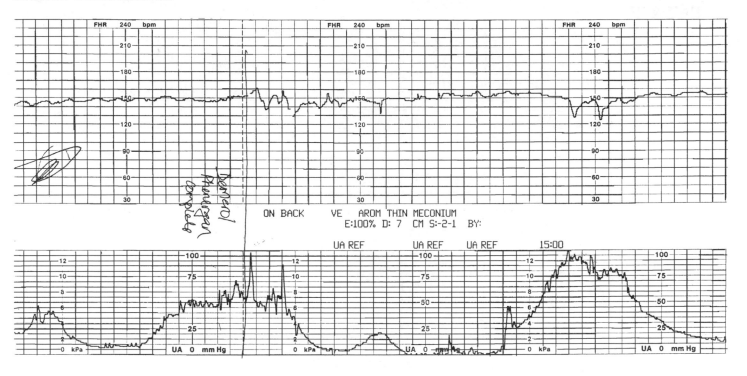

4.11   Tetanic contractions are long and strong (≥ 90 seconds x ≥ 90 mm Hg).

Tetanic contractions are long and strong, i.e., they usually last 90 or more seconds, are strong to palpation and reach or exceed 90 mm Hg. Tetanic contractions can occur during normal labors. If they do, expect rapid labor progress. However, they can also occur as a response to cocaine. Cocaine causes the release of oxytocin from the posterior pituitary gland and also has a direct effect on uterine cells.

Uterine Irritability

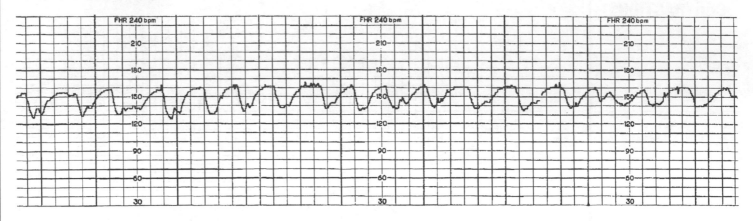

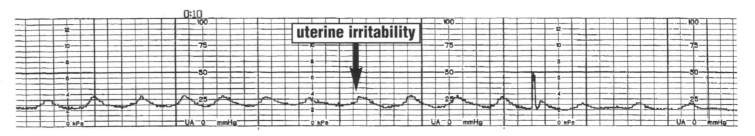

*4.12   LAHF waves or uterine irritability and a rarely seen series of accelerations that look like a
sinusoidal pattern. The fetus eventually had a baseline of 120-130 bpm.*

Low amplitude high frequency waves (LAHF waves), or uterine irritability, is often related to uterine prostaglandin release which results from infection or the lack of adequate uterine perfusion due to dehydration. If the
woman is preterm, LAHF waves may occur in the 72 hours preceding the onset of preterm labor. Some women
have LAHF waves when the placenta is abrupting.

Exercises

For each example, describe the frequency, duration, strength, and relaxation or resting tone.

4.

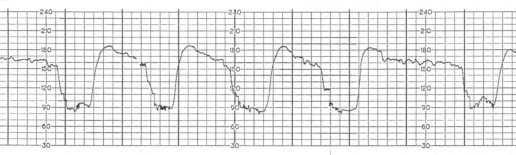

4.13 *Variable decelerations with overshoots. Uterine activity pattern demonstrates maternal respirations and contractions.*

Frequency _____

Duration _____

Strength _____

Resting Tone _____

5.

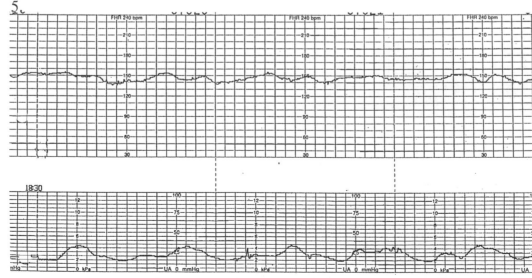

4.14 *Abruption. Absent long-term and short-term variability.*

Frequency _____

Duration _____

Strength _____

Resting Tone _____

6.

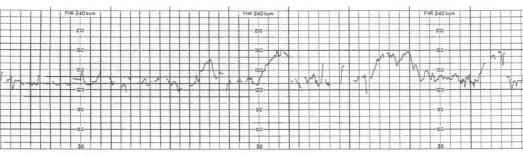

4.15 *Ultrasound and tocotransducer used. Confirm uterine activity by palpation. Adjust TOCO as required.*

Frequency _____

Duration _____

Strength _____

Resting Tone _____

7.

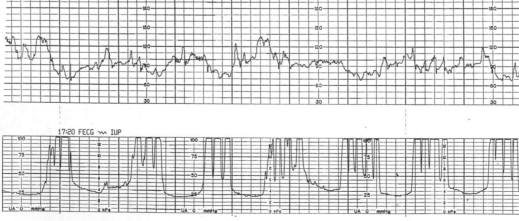

4.16 *Pushing with second-stage (end-stage) bradycardia.*

Frequency _____

Duration _____

Strength _____

Resting Tone _____

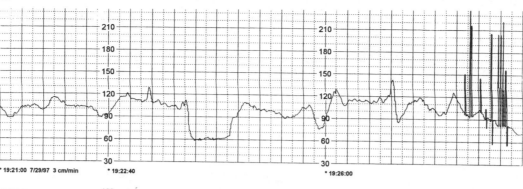

4.17 **Computer printout of a fetal monitor tracing. Unstable FHR, variable decelerations and artifact.**

Frequency _____

Duration _____

Strength _____

Resting Tone _____

ANSWERS TO EXERCISES

1. 200 MVUs

2. 105 MVUs

3. 185 MVUs

4. q 1¹/₂ -2¹/₂ minutes x 40-70 seconds, need to palpate strength and resting tone [q means every]

5. hyperstimulation, approximately q 1¹/₂ minutes x 30-70 seconds, need to palpate strength. The placenta is abrupting. This is a medical emergency.

6. no uterine activity. Fetal or maternal movement spikes only.

7. hyperstimulation, occasional hypertonus, q 1¹/₂ minutes x 50-70, strong (pushing), need to palpate resting tone and act to decrease uterine activity.

8. q 1¹/₂ -2 minutes, 50-80, pushing then panting, palpate resting tone, act to facilitate delivery.

SUMMARY

Summary

Contraction frequency often increases when the woman is fearful and anxious. Frequency, duration, strength, and relaxation are documented when the uterus is palpated or a tocotransducer is used. Frequency, duration, peak intrauterine pressure, and resting tone are documented when an intrauterine pressure catheter is used.

Montevideo units (MVUs) are calculated by adding contraction intensities over a 10 minute period. Intensity is the contraction peak minus its resting tone. Intensity can only be measured when an intrauterine pressure catheter is in place. 150 or more MVUs have been associated with adequate labor progress.

Dystocia is associated with abnormally slow or no cervical change. Often, the presenting part is not well applied to the cervix. Reduction of a woman's fear, oxytocin augmentation, hydration, or narcotics may improve uterine contraction effectiveness.

Contractions appear in sets (coupling) when the fetus is in a persistent occiput posterior or occiput transverse position. Hyperstimulation may be related to Pitocin® hypersensitivity, prostaglandin or cocaine use, or placental abruption. Hyperstimulation syndrome exists when there is an abnormal fetal heart rate related to uterine hyperstimulation. Hypertonus is a resting tone greater than 25 mm Hg. Uterine reversal appears when the tocotransducer is not placed above the umbilicus at term or the abdomen moves away from it during a contraction. Tetanic contractions suggest rapid labor progress, imminent delivery, or a response to cocaine. Uterine irritability or low amplitude high frequency waves suggest prostaglandin release due to infection, dehydration with a lack of uterine perfusion, abruption, or impending preterm labor.

SECTION 4: UTERINE CONTRACTIONS

QUESTIONS

Directions: Circle T if the statement is true, F if it is false.

QUESTIONS

T   F

T   F

T   F

T   F

T   F

T   F

T   F

T   F

T   F

T   F

1.   Fear decreases uterine activity.

2.   A resting tone of 8 to 12 mm Hg is normal.

3.   The interval is the time from the beginning of one contraction to the beginning of the next contraction.

4.   Intensity, or active pressure, is synonymous with strength or quality of contractions.

5.   Calculation of Montevideo Units should be used to identify hypocontractility.

6.   Abnormal labor may be related to a fetal presenting part that is not well applied to the cervix.

7.   A tocotransducer can provide fairly accurate information on contraction frequency and duration.

8.   Contraction detection with a tocotransducer in a preterm gestation is as accurate as in a term gestation.

9.   An intrauterine pressure catheter is needed to evaluate peak intrauterine pressure.

10.   An occiput posterior position is related to uterine contraction coupling.

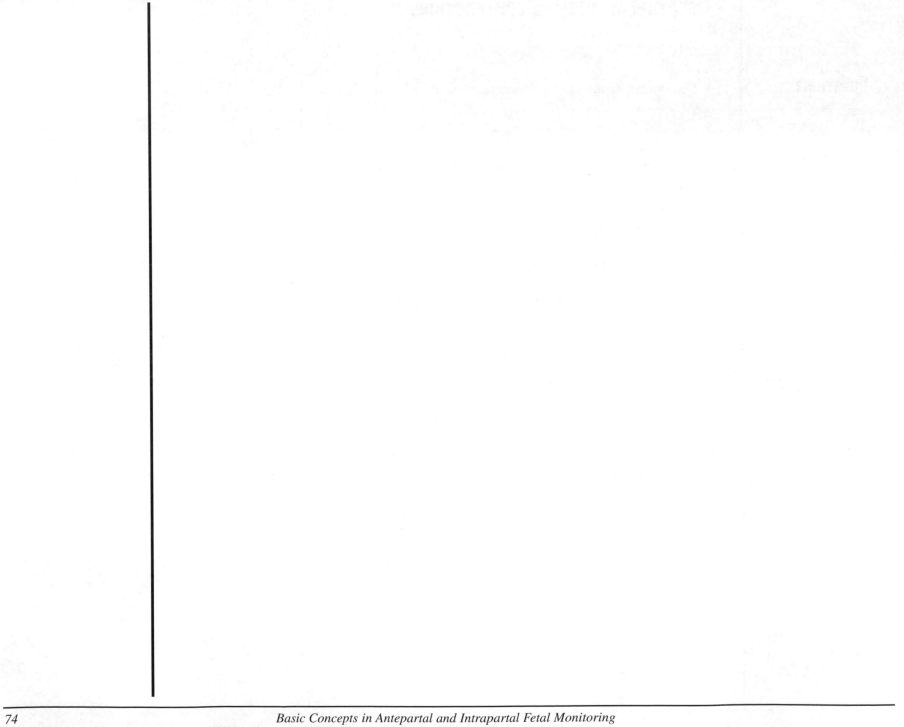

SECTION 5
The Baseline (BL)

A systematic review of the fetal heart rate (FHR) includes the determination of the baseline, accelerations (accels), and decelerations (decels). A FHR pattern is a combination of BL, accels, and decels. There is actually no time limit for determining a BL rate. In fact, a flat baseline will be obvious in one minute e.g., a persistent rate of 150 beats per minute (bpm).

In addition to a baseline, accels, and decels, you may see artifact or suspect a dysrhythmia. With practice, it becomes easier to identify:

* the baseline

* accelerations

* decelerations

* artifact

* dysrhythmia and

* maternal heart rate patterns.

Some clinicians learned they need to see 10 minutes of tracing to determine a baseline. Others need just one or two minutes. Look at figure 5.1. You will see a baseline and accelerations.

Scan the tracing in figure 5.1. The baseline is fluctuating yet considered to be stable between 122 and 135 bpm. The baseline may rise as a result of fetal hypoxia or an increase in maternal temperature. The baseline may abruptly or gradually flatten and decrease as a result of fetal decompensation. Figure 5.1 has neither a rising nor falling baseline.

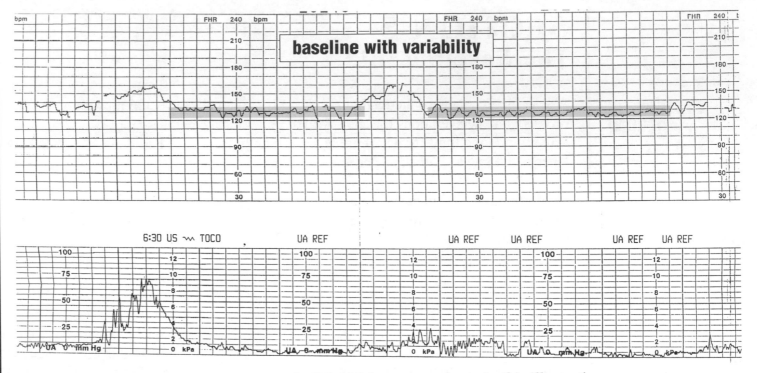

5.1 *The FHR baseline is approximately 122-135 beats per minute in this illustration.*

Baseline Physiology

The baseline is the FHR created primarily by the influence of the vagus and sympathetic nerves on the heart. The baseline is also influenced by hormonal and pharmacologic factors. For example, fetal catecholamines may cause a rise in the baseline level, or fetal arginine vasopressin (antidiuretic hormone) may cause a sinusoidal baseline. Narcotics may flatten a baseline or create a benign sinusoidal pattern. Fetuses spend an average of 23 minutes and no more than 100 minutes at a time in a quiet sleep. This behavioral state is accompanied by a stable but flat or nearly flat baseline.

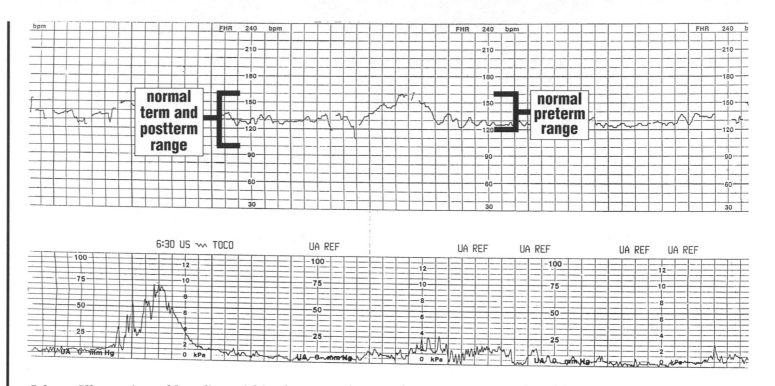

5.2   *Illustration of baseline within the normal range for a term or postterm fetus.*

The baseline is approximately 122-135 bpm. The normal baseline will lie between 100-160 bpm for term and postterm fetuses and 120-160 bpm for preterm fetuses. The baseline should be at a similar level from 35 weeks to delivery. If the fetus is oxygenated, the baseline may move within a 20 bpm range.

Variability

Variability is a baseline characteristic and is also called long-term variability. It is not an acceleration or deceleration. Variability is present when the baseline is chaotic, irregular and fluctuating. Variability is absent when the baseline is regular, nonchaotic, and/or smooth. Long-term variability includes cycles. One cycle looks like this:

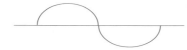

A series of cycles creates long-term variability. When long-term variability is present there usually will be 2 or more cycles per minute. Section 6 discusses classifications of long-term variability.

Another characteristic of the baseline is short-term variability. Section 7 discusses short-term variability.

Long-term variability should **not** be interpreted as reassuring unless accelerations are also present within the last 100 minutes of monitoring. Acute hypoxia may abruptly increase long-term variability. Causes of acute hypoxia include cord compression, uterine hyperstimulation, and maternal hypotension. The baseline range will be greater than 25 bpm with acute hypoxia.

Chronic hypoxia, with the accumulation of adenosine from the anaerobic metabolism of adenosine triphosphate, decreases long-term variability and the baseline flattens.

THE LOSS OF VARIABILITY/ FLAT BASELINE

The loss of variability may be caused by drugs such as narcotics. A flat baseline may be worse than a baseline with decelerations, particularly when the lack of variability is related to fetal metabolic acidosis. By obtaining a detailed history and reviewing clinical events, such as narcotic administration, the presence of maternal infection or meconium, and fetal movement, you may be able to determine the cause of absent variability.

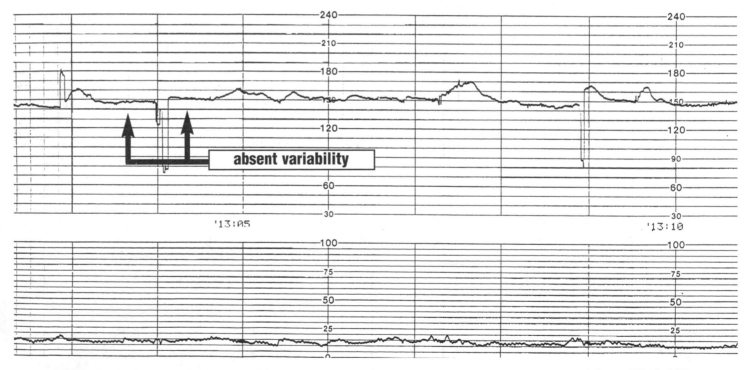

5.3 *Baseline of 148-152 beats per minute with spontaneous accelerations to 160-170 bpm. Variability may be decreased due to Tegretol® and Prozac®. However, there is no research to confirm the effect of these drugs on the fetal heart rate. Fetal movement is present. Apgars were 7 and 9 at 1 and 5 minutes.*

Beta-blockers, such as Tenormin® (atenolol) decrease long-term variability and accelerations.

Persistent absent variability (greater than 100 minutes), or a flat baseline, may be due to direct myocardial depression as a result of metabolic acidosis. Over the course of two days and a prolonged labor, the fetus progressively deteriorated and was born asphyxiated (see 5.4 and 5.5).

RISING BASELINE

The baseline may flatten, and/or rise over a period of minutes or hours, while accelerations disappear. At 1100, the baseline was 120-122 bpm (see 5.4). By noon, it was over 150 bpm with prolonged decelerations (see 5.5). The flattening and/or rising baseline is a response to hypoxia. By itself, a rising baseline is classified as compensatory. When you add one or more prolonged decelerations, the FHR pattern becomes nonreassuring. Hypoxic fetuses reduce their movement. Notify the midwife or physician when a rising baseline occurs. Assess fetal movement by palpation and/or ask the woman when her baby moved last. Take the maternal temperature and pulse and rule out uterine tenderness. When was the last acceleration? If the membranes have ruptured, note the color, amount, and odor of the amniotic fluid. Chorioamnionitis is related to hypoxia and a rising baseline.

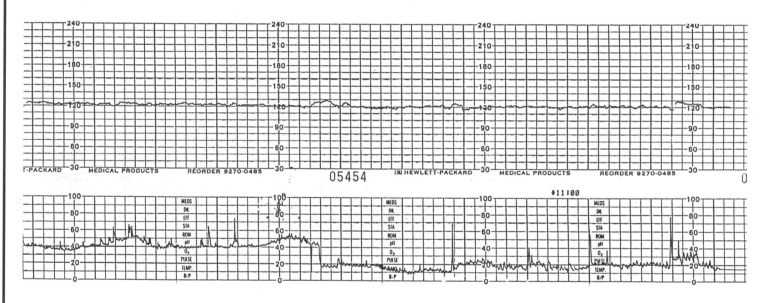

5.4   Initial baseline was 120-122 bpm.

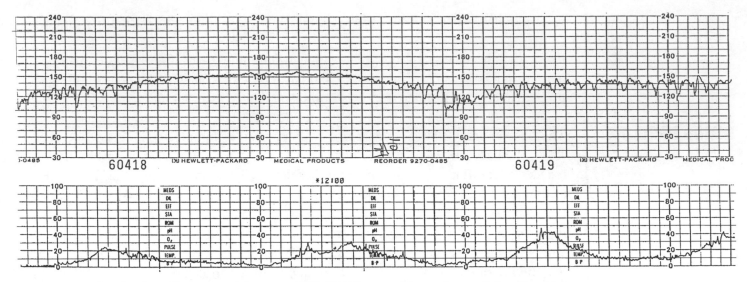

5.5   *Rise in the baseline over 1 hour to 150-155 bpm with prolonged decelerations.*

A tachycardic FHR is a rate greater than 160 bpm. This is abnormal and may be a response to hypoxia. Identify and document the maternal temperature, pulse, uterine tenderness, and color, amount, and odor of amniotic fluid. Note any accelerations, fetal movement, and short-term variability. Notify the midwife or physician when tachycardia lasts 10 or more minutes.

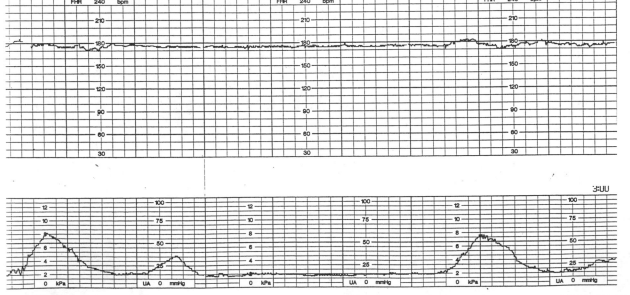

5.6 Tachycardia is defined by a FHR baseline greater than 160 bpm. In this strip the baseline average is 175 bpm.

BRADYCARDIA (TERM, POST TERM)

The definition of bradycardia varies with fetal gestation. A rate less than 100 bpm would be bradycardic if the fetus is mature (≥ 38 weeks of gestation). A rate between 100 and 120 bpm is normal in a term or postterm fetus due to their large heart and mature nervous system. To reassure yourself that this is a normal rate and rhythm, identify and document accelerations and fetal movement. A preterm FHR less than 120 bpm is bradycardic.

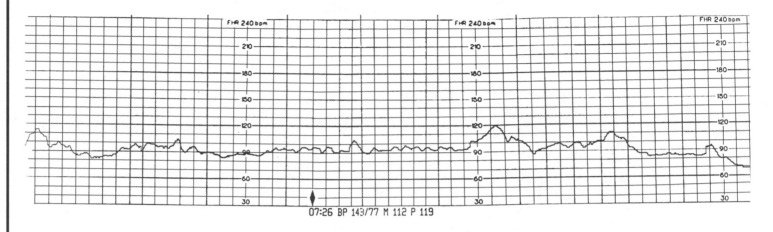

07:26 BP 143/77 M 112 P 119

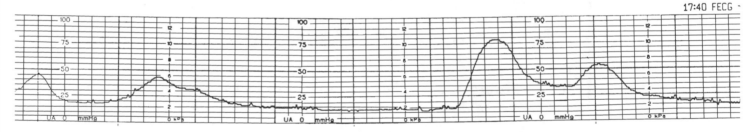

17:40 FECG

5.7 *Bradycardia is a baseline less than 100 bpm in a term or postterm fetus. The baseline is 90-100 bpm. This baby was 39 weeks of gestation. Note the spontaneous accelerations. This is a non-acidotic fetus who has bradycardia. Also note the coupling of contractions prior to 1740 and the maternal blood pressure of 143/77, mean arterial pressure of 112, and heart rate of 119 bpm. Could this fetus be occiput posterior with head compression (producing a vagal response and bradycardia)? Notify the midwife or physician of fetal bradycardia.*

A baseline less than 120 bpm is bradycardia if the fetus is preterm.

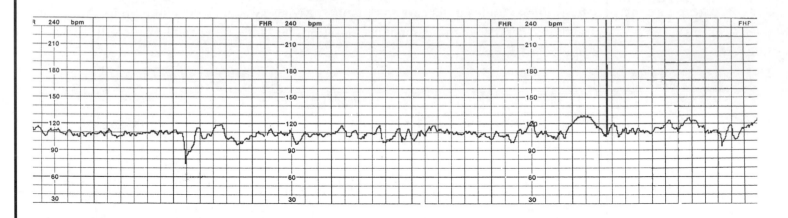

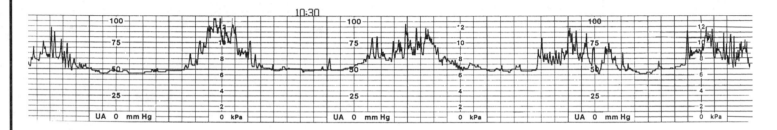

5.8   *Preterm bradycardia at 37 weeks of gestation. Is it possible that this is a term fetus and the estimated date of delivery (EDD) is not correct? To lower the uterine activity waveform, press the "UA" button.*

A falling baseline may occur abruptly or slowly. The fetus needs to be evaluated immediately. If there are no accelerations and a loss of variability, or the baseline continues to fall, the pattern requires immediate medical attention by both an obstetrician and anesthesia provider.

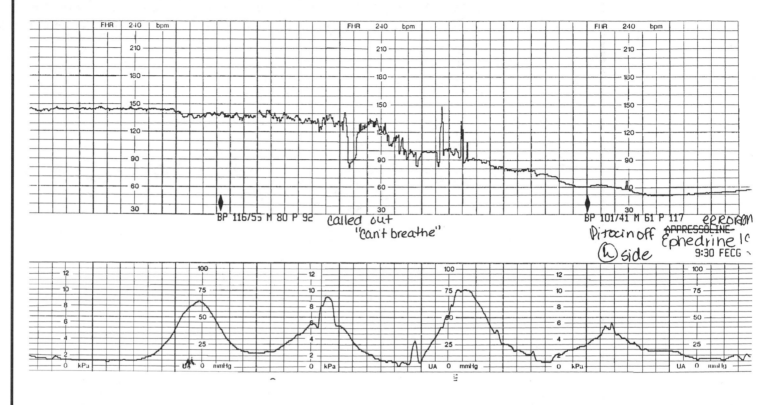

5.9 *Falling baseline due to a "high" spinal. This baby had Apgars of 0 at 1, 5, and 10 minutes. The cord artery pH was 6.4. Note the uterine hyperstimulation and the maternal respiratory distress. A hypoxic uterus releases prostaglandins which causes uterine hyperstimulation. Ephedrine is given by slow IV push to increase blood pressure. Note the blood pressure dropped from 116/55 to 101/41.*

WANDERING BASELINE

A wandering baseline is a smooth, meandering FHR with absent variability. It is considered to be unstable and ominous because it is usually associated with fetal asphyxia. Sometimes the baseline rate will move between rates that are 40 or more bpm apart. It never stabilizes. Measures to enhance fetal oxygenation should be instituted immediately, and delivery should be expedited, especially if congenital anomalies have been ruled out by a previous ultrasound. A pediatrician and/or neonatal resusitation team should attend the delivery.

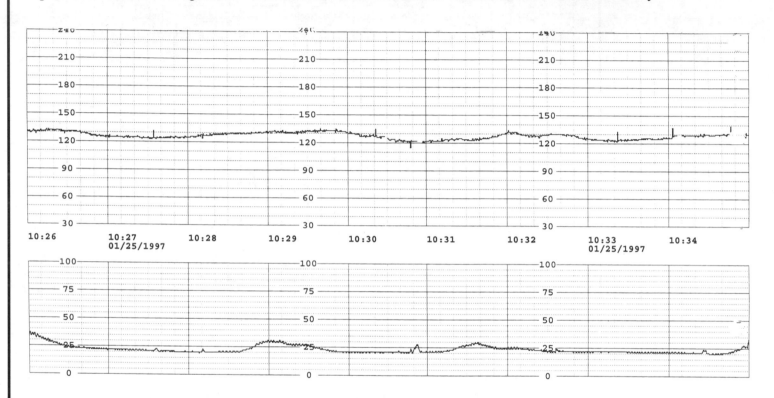

5.10   A wandering baseline may be a reflection of fetal asphyxiation and rarely is seen with a brain or congenital anomaly.

AGONAL PATTERN

Agonal patterns are bradycardia usually related to cord compression, such as cord prolapse. The fetus is anoxic and unable to maintain its heart rate. The upward surge of the FHR is due to epinephrine and norepinephrine (catecholamines) from the fetal adrenal glands. In spite of this response, there is fetal decompensation with complete cardiovascular collapse. The FHR is ominous and demands immediate delivery and resuscitation. Document the rate, e.g., "60-100, 0 STV, 0 LTV." Rule out a cord prolapse and assess dilatation. Can she push the baby out? Call the obstetrician, anesthesia provider, and pediatrician/neonatal resuscitation team stat. It is not appropriate to waste time or delay delivery with position changes or other measures to enhance oxygen delivery to the fetus unless the surgeon is not immediately available. Scalp stimulation is inappropriate because it is an assessment technique to evoke FHR accelerations to rule out metabolic acidosis. Abdominal (external) manipulation has no effect on the fetus. Oxygen at 8 to 10 liters per minute via a simple tight fitting face mask or a 500 ml intravenous bolus of lactated Ringer's solution may have little impact on fetal oxygenation and uterine activity. Discontinue oxytocics. A tocolytic, such as terbutaline, may decrease uterine activity. Terbutaline is contraindicated if there is a placental abruption.

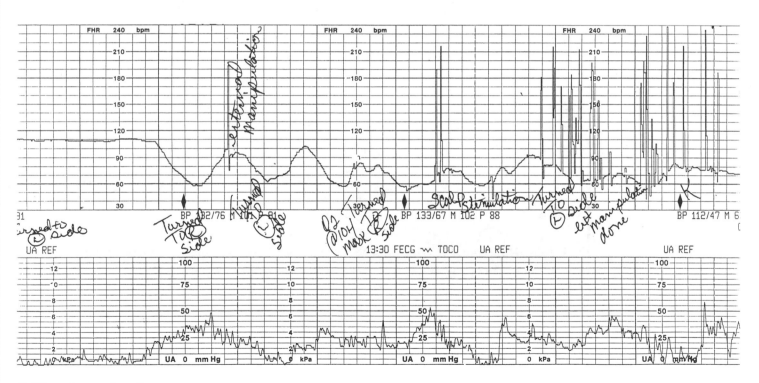

5.11   Agonal pattern.

The baseline is documented as an average rate, e.g., 135 bpm, or as a range, e.g., 130s or 130-140 bpm. If the baseline is not exactly a 10 bpm range, do not generalize. Instead, be specific, e.g., 132-136. It is recommended to utilize the baseline range method in nursing notes because 5 percent of tracings are lost or are missing in actual lawsuits. From your note, the FHR pattern could be recreated. By being specific, a clear image of what you observed is created in the reader's mind.

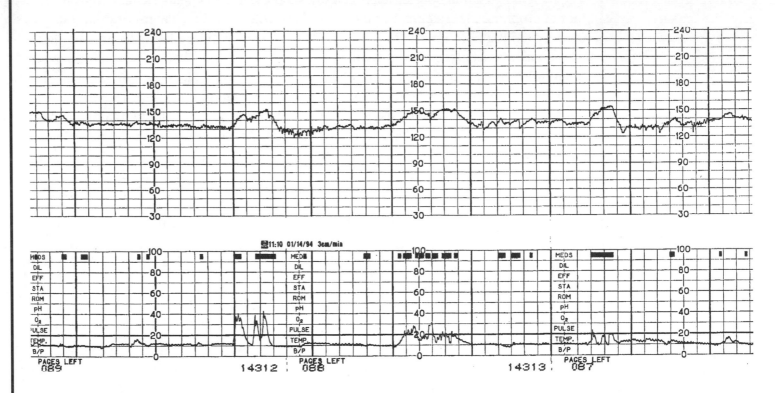

5.12　*Baseline 130-140 bpm. Also note spontaneous accelerations, spikes reflective of fetal movement, and fetal movement marks at the top of the uterine activity channel. This tracing reflects a nonacidotic, nonasphyxiated fetus.*

TERMINAL BRADYCARDIA

An ominous FHR pattern demanding delivery and resuscitation is terminal bradycardia. Note the absence of variability. The FHR is mostly less than 80 bpm and falling. Document the rate, e.g., 70 bpm, 0 STV, 0 LTV. Call the surgeon, anesthesia provider, and pediatrician/neonatal resusitation team stat.

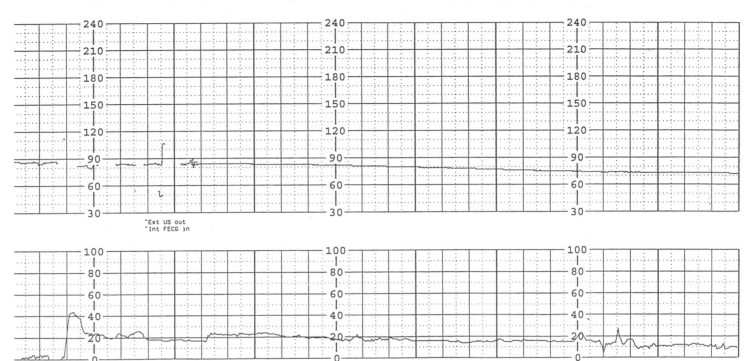

5.13 *Terminal bradycardia in a primigravida at 40 weeks of gestation. Apgars 1, 3, and 6 at 1, 5, and 10 minutes.*

Actions in Response to an Agonal Pattern and Terminal Bradycardia

- mobilize all available personnel

- prepare for cesarean section if vaginal delivery is not imminent

- prepare for neonatal resuscitation

- call stat:

  - "any available obstetrician" if the attending physician or surgeon is not in the hospital

  - anesthesia provider

  - neonatal resuscitation team, including a physician or neonatal nurse practitioner who can manage neonatal complications, including intubation and drug administration

- act to improve fetal oxygenation, although this may not change the FHR pattern

- prepare the woman for delivery, which may include minimal preparations for a cesarean section, e.g., a foley catheter

- ask family members to wait in the waiting room

- if personnel are available, a member of the health care team should stay with the family and explain events

- deliver the fetus as soon as the team is mobilized.

END-STAGE BRADYCARDIA

End-stage, Second-stage, or Birth Bradycardia

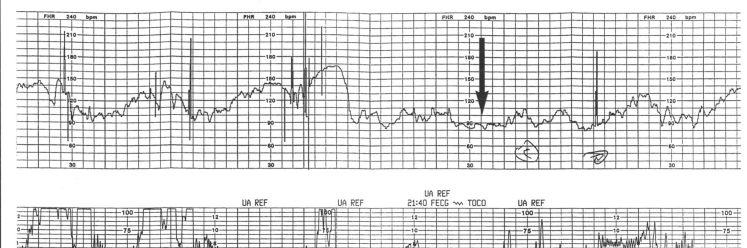

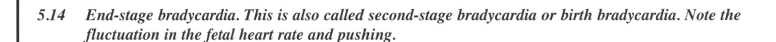

5.14   End-stage bradycardia. This is also called second-stage bradycardia or birth bradycardia. Note the fluctuation in the fetal heart rate and pushing.

End-stage bradycardia is a compensatory pattern that often precedes a vaginal birth. During the minutes before birth when the head and cord are compressed, the baseline drops an average of 45 bpm, but long-term variability is average to moderate and accelerations occasionally appear. Variable decelerations or a prolonged deceleration might appear but short-term variability is present. **As long as the FHR is greater than 90 bpm and delivery will occur** *in a few minutes***, supplemental oxygen is not needed**. Document the bpm, e.g., "80-90 bpm." It is optional to write end-stage or second-stage bradycardia. These fetuses are usually born needing no more than stimulation, e.g., dry them off, or you may need to provide brief blow-by oxygen. **The longer the rate is less than 90 bpm, the greater the risk for fetal acidemia**. If you wait to begin pushing until the woman feels the urge, there will be less risk of fetal bradycardia.

SUMMARY

Summary

A systematic review of the fetal heart rate pattern includes assessment of the baseline, accelerations,.and decelerations. There may also be artifact and/or you may suspect a dysrhythmia. The baseline can be assessed in one to two minutes, especially if it is flat. The baseline fluctuations are caused by vagal and sympathetic nerve influences and may also be influenced by fetal hormones or drugs. Variability, as a general concept, refers to the chaotic, irregular fluctuations in the baseline and consists of 2 or more cycles per minute. Acute hypoxia may create a baseline range greater than 25 bpm (marked or saltatory long-term variability). The loss of variability may be due to hypoxia, narcotics or beta-blockers. Variability is only reassuring if accelerations are present within 100 minutes of monitoring. Persistent absent variability may be due to metabolic acidosis.

Alterations in the baseline, such as a rising baseline, suggest a compensatory response to hypoxia and can be found with chorioamnionitis. Tachycardia is a rate greater than 160 bpm. A falling baseline suggests fetal decompensation. A wandering baseline is usually related to fetal asphyxia and is rarely related to a congenital defect.

Bradycardia in a term or postterm fetus is a rate less than 100 bpm. Bradycardia in a preterm fetus is a rate less than 120 bpm. An agonal pattern and terminal bradycardia suggest a high risk for asphyxia and death. Once a fetus has a terminal or agonal pattern or bradycardia, it does not spontaneously recover. Therefore, the goal is to deliver and resuscitate.

An agonal pattern is a fetal bradycardia that lacks variability, but has upward and downward swings in the fetal heart rate caused by fetal catecholamine release. It is ominous and a predeath pattern. Agonal patterns are often related to cord compression, e.g., due to cord prolapse. The immediate goal is to deliver and resuscitate.

End-stage, second-stage, or birth bradycardia is common prior to vaginal delivery, and is caused by head and cord compression. Since variability and accelerations persist, expect a good outcome. However, the longer the rate is less than 90 bpm, the greater the risk of fetal acidemia becomes.

SECTION 5: THE BASELINE

QUESTIONS

Directions: Circle T if the statement is true, F if it is false.

QUESTIONS

T   F

T   F

T   F

T   F

T   F

T   F

T   F

T   F

T   F

T   F

1. A systematic review of the fetal heart rate includes the baseline, accelerations, and decelerations.

2. The baseline has cycles.

3. A baseline is determined only after a review of 10 minutes of the tracing.

4. The baseline is influenced by neural, nutritional, hormonal and pharmacologic factors.

5. Fetal heart rate baseline changes can occur abruptly or over minutes.

6. Preterm infants have a normal heart rate range between 100 and 160 beats per minute.

7. Variability is a baseline characteristic.

8. A rising or falling baseline may indicate hypoxia.

9. The baseline of an asphyxiated fetus has variability.

10. A wandering baseline requires actions to improve fetal oxygenation and expedite delivery.

SECTION 6
Long-Term Variability (LTV)

In Section 5 you identified the fetal heart rate (FHR) baseline. In this section you will learn to identify long-term variability (LTV). **LTV is a baseline characteristic** and is not evaluated during a deceleration or acceleration.

SINE WAVE, OSCILLATION, CYCLE, COMPLEX

As each consecutive FHR is determined and printed, the baseline appears to rise and fall creating small, crude undulations or waves around the average rate. This is long-term variability (LTV). One wave is also called a sine wave, oscillation, cycle, or complex. Most oxygenated fetuses have 2 to 8 cycles per minute (cpm). Determine the cycle amplitude of the baseline prior to categorizing LTV.

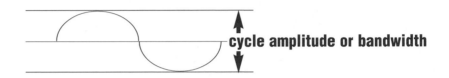

1 cycle, sine wave, oscillation, or complex

Documentation of Cycles

BANDWIDTH

AMPLITUDE/ RANGE

Although LTV is observed as cycles per minute, it is not documented as such. Instead, LTV is classified and documented based on the bpm range between the top and bottom of the majority of cycles. This range is called the *bandwidth*. It is usually similar to the baseline range especially when the baseline is stable. The bandwidth is also called the *amplitude* of the baseline.

CLASSIFICATION OF LTV BASED ON AMPLITUDE

Over the years, several systems have been developed to document LTV observations. In fact, LTV may fluctuate between a narrow bandwidth, e.g., 3 bpm, to a wider bandwidth, e.g., 25 bpm or more. Therefore, it is usual to document more than one category of LTV. Determine the top of most of the cycles, the bottom of most of the cycles, and then calculate the bpm between these two levels.

Five categories of LTV are listed with their bandwidth range.

LTV Category	Bandwidth Range
absent	0 - 2 bpm or ≤ 1¹/₂ cpm
minimal or decreased	3 - 5 bpm
average	6 - 10 bpm
moderate	11 - 25 bpm
marked, saltatory, or increased	> 25 bpm

LTV in and of itself is not the only predictor of fetal well-being. **However, the absence of LTV may reflect fetal compromise, especially if there have been no accelerations for 100 or more minutes**. Identify the last acceleration. Is there short-term variability? Your facility may not use all 5 categories to document LTV.

To judge the quality of your documentation ask, "Could I draw the pattern from what I charted?" Accuracy in charting LTV helps recreate the tracing if it is lost.

ABSENT LTV

Absent LTV

Most babies have average to moderate LTV most of the time. Absent LTV is less than or equal to 1¹/₂ cycles per minute or a baseline with a range of 0 to 2 bpm (flat or nearly flat). Absent LTV often is related to depressant drugs, such as narcotics. It can also occur during fetal quiet sleep (quiescent fetal state) which lasts an average of 23 minutes in near-term or term fetuses. However, it may last up to 100 minutes.

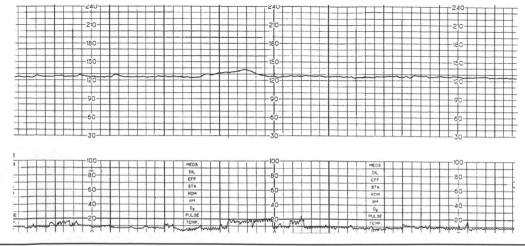

6.1   Illustration of long-term variability that is absent to minimal. Magnesium sulfate (6 gm bolus) may be associated with the loss of LTV. However a well baby will still accelerate.

Essentials of Fetal Monitoring

CAUSES OF ABSENT LTV

Cause(s)/Physiology of Absent LTV

- fetal quiescent state or quiet sleep (also known as the 1F state)

- drugs, e.g., narcotics, cigarettes, and cocaine

- hypoxia

- severe fetal anemia, e.g., as a result of a fetal viral infection

- dysrhythmia such as supraventricular tachycardia or complete heart block

- cardiovascular lesions or chromosomal aberration, often accompanied by variable decels and bradycardia.

- fetal brain death or decerebration

- congenital brain anomaly, e.g., anencephaly with only spinal cord function

- cerebral ischemia.

Absent LTV is also a late sign of deterioration of the intrauterine growth restricted fetus. *Bradycardia and absent LTV, i.e., terminal bradycardia, not related to a dysrhythmia, suggests impending intrauterine death.*

ACTIONS WHEN LTV IS ABSENT

Actions When LTV is Absent

Absent LTV is nonreassuring until the cause is determined. Actions to determine the significance of absent LTV include obtaining a fetal movement history, assessing fetal movement by palpation or real-time ultrasound, and reviewing the tracing to determine if there have been any accelerations in the last 60 to 100 minutes. Obtain a maternal drug use history. Apply a spiral electrode to assess short-term variability. Note the presence or absence of meconium in the amniotic fluid and notify the midwife or physician promptly if you cannot find a sign of fetal well-being.

WANDERING BASELINE WITH ABSENT LTV

One cycle per minute is abnormal and reflects absent LTV. Absent LTV in the non-narcotized fetus is usually indicative of fetal metabolic acidosis, asphyxia, or neurologic damage. A wandering baseline (with absent LTV) should be immediately reported to the obstetrician. If a congenital defect does not exist, act to increase fetal oxygenation and expedite delivery. A pediatrician and resusitation team should attend the delivery.

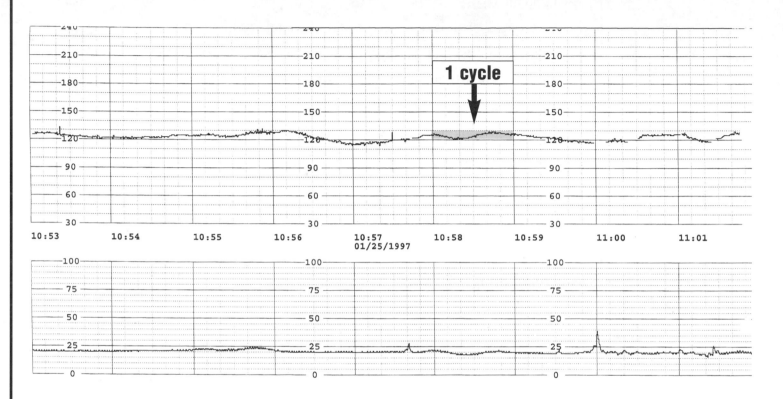

6.2   A wandering baseline with less than 1½ cycles per minute or absent long-term variability.

Minimal LTV

Minimal LTV (3 to 5 beats per minutes bandwidth) may occur when the fetus is in a quiet sleep state or has a narcotic "on board." Minimal LTV may also represent a lack of oxygen, or hypoxia. To differentiate hypoxia from a quiet sleep state or a medication effect, examine the fetal heart rate tracing 60 minutes prior to the "minimal" LTV. Do you see accelerations? Review the nurses' notes for drug administration. Determine the probable cause of minimal LTV.

Cause(s)/Physiology of Minimal LTV (3-5 bpm)

Alternative Label: decreased LTV

Minimal LTV may be present when the fetus has:

• a temperature elevation (tachycardia will be present too)

• hypovolemia, hypoxia, or acidosis (tachycardia may be present too)

• a central nervous system depressant "on board"

• moved into a quiescent (1F) state.

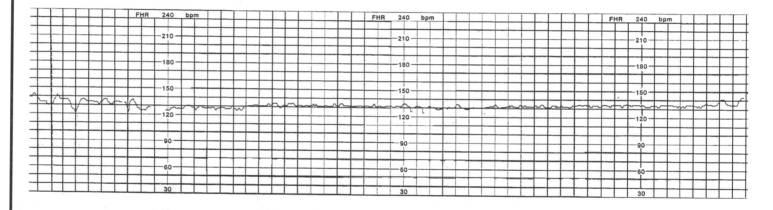

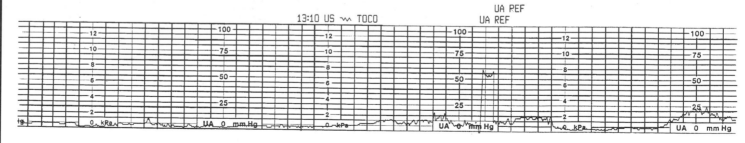

6.3   Minimal long-term variability.

Average LTV

Average LTV is a normal finding and represents integrity of the sympathetic and parasympathetic (vagus) nervous systems. There is adequate oxygen delivery to the brainstem. There should also be spontaneous accelerations and fetal movement. A pathological sinusoidal pattern may have average LTV but there will be decreased or no fetal movement, no accelerations, and decreased or absent short-term variability.

Cause(s)/Physiology of Average LTV (6-10 bpm):

- neural integrity when accompanied by accelerations and fetal movement.

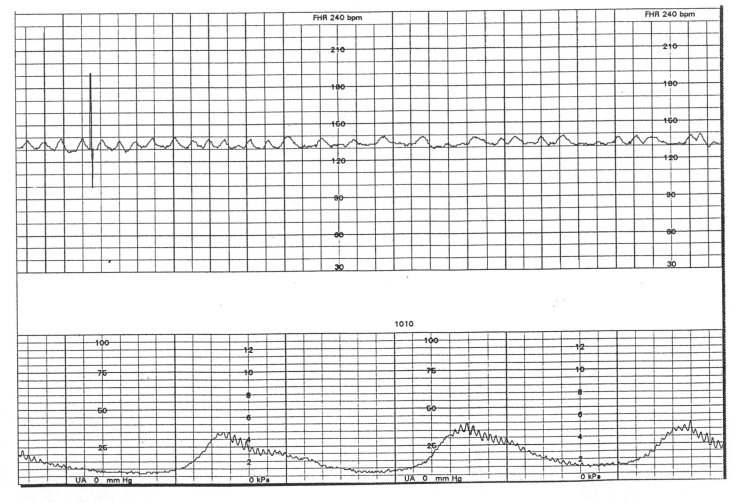

6.4   *Average long-term variability.*

Essentials of Fetal Monitoring

MODERATE LTV

Moderate LTV is normal. Moderate LTV is seen when there are accelerations and fetal movement. However, it may be a response to Ephedrine® administration, vacuum extractor application, or a slight decrease in oxygenation.

Cause(s)/Physiology of Moderate LTV (11-25 bpm):

- active sleep (2F) or active awake (4F) state of fetus

- application of the vacuum extractor (may also see marked LTV)

- maternal Ephedrine® to correct hypotension (may also see marked LTV).

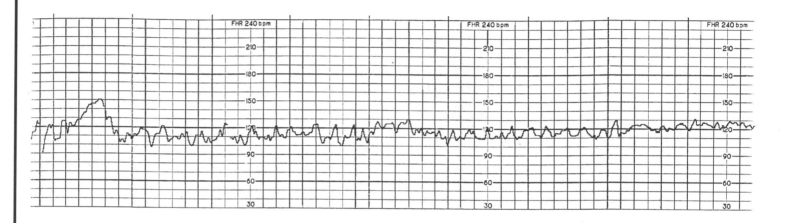

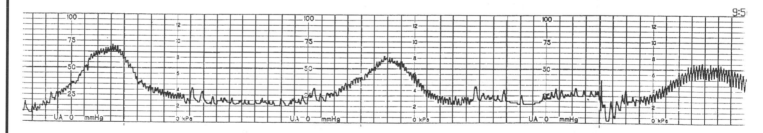

6.5   Moderate long-term variability following a spontaneous acceleration. Note the fluctuation of the baseline within a 20 bpm range (100-120).

Some clinicians have labeled a baseline bandwidth of 6 to 25 bpm as average long-term variability. This is one way to collapse two categories into one. However, if the baseline range is not near 25 bpm, and the strip is lost, the tracing will be difficult to recreate.

MARKED OR SALTATORY LTV

Marked LTV, also called a saltatory pattern or saltatory baseline, usually suggests an **acute** fetal compensatory response to a hypoxic event, such as umbilical cord compression, uterine hyperstimulation, or maternal hypotension. A saltatory pattern is a chaotic, jumping baseline with a cycle bandwidth of more than 25 bpm. It may be preceded by a variable or prolonged deceleration. It may also follow maternal hypotension and Ephedrine® administration. Actions to improve fetal oxygenation must be taken, such as a maternal position change, a 500 ml intravenous bolus with a non-glucose solution such as lactated Ringer's, and hyperoxygenation with a face mask. If a simple mask is used, set the oxygen flow to 8 or more liters per minute. If a partial rebreathing mask is used, set the flow at 12 liters per minute to prevent carbon dioxide from entering the oxygen reservoir.

HYPER-OXYGENATION BENEFITS

The benefits of maternal oxygen administration include:

- increased fetal brain oxygen

- improved fetal circulation

- increased fetal PaO_2

- increased fetal SaO_2

- increased fetal tissue O_2

- increased fetal breathing movements

- increased fetal body movements

- reappearance of accelerations

- improved variability

- decrease or absense of late decelerations

- fewer neonatal resuscitations.

Oxygen should reach the fetus by the 10th minute after oxygen initiation. If the FHR pattern does not improve within 20 minutes, oxygen delivery may be impeded. The midwife or physician may need to consider expediting delivery. Therefore, it is important to let them know your assessments, actions, and the maternal and fetal responses within 10 to 15 minutes of initiating actions to improve fetal oxygenation.

Essentials of Fetal Monitoring

Marked LTV

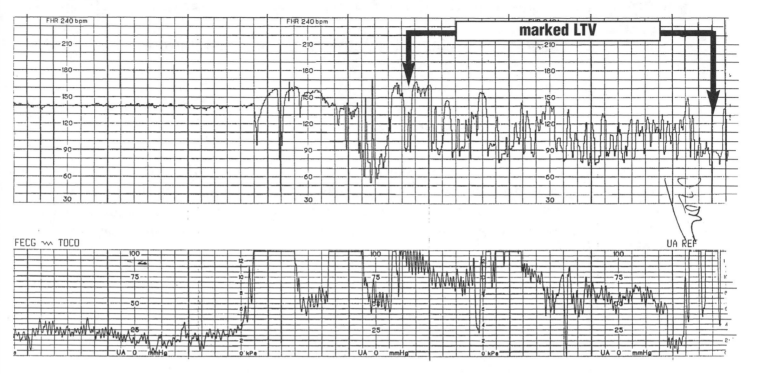

6.6   *In this strip the long-term variability (LTV) changed from absent to marked near the time of delivery due to cord compression and acute hypoxia.*

Cause(s)/Physiology of Marked LTV:

- if noted when an ultrasound transducer is used, may be caused by a fetal dysrhythmia such as premature ventricular contractions

- rare in preterm fetuses

- high incidence in postterm fetuses, possibly due to neurologic maturation

- usually a compensatory response to a hypoxic event, e.g., umbilical cord compression or uterine hyperstimulation

- may follow Ephedrine® administration for hypotension

- may be observed during the second stage of labor, especially with use of the vacuum extractor.

A series of sine waves creates a *sinusoidal pattern or sinusoidal baseline*. Sinusoidal patterns may represent a *pathological* process such as fetal hypoxia, acidosis, or asphyxia.

Cause(s)/Physiology of a Pathologic Sinusoidal Pattern:

- hypoxia related to:
  Rh disease (erythroblastosis fetalis) with hemolysis/anemia,
  cord compression, infection, preclampsia, abruption, fetal hypovolemia
- acidosis or asphyxia.

Some clinicians think a sinusoidal pattern differs from variability, but they are essentially the same thing. The sinusoidal pattern is also called a sinusoidal baseline. It has smooth, or nearly smooth cycles, with a similar frequency and amplitude. Cycles are a baseline characteristic. A sinusoidal pattern may be pathologic or benign. Benign sinusoidal patterns are also called physiologic sinusoidal patterns.

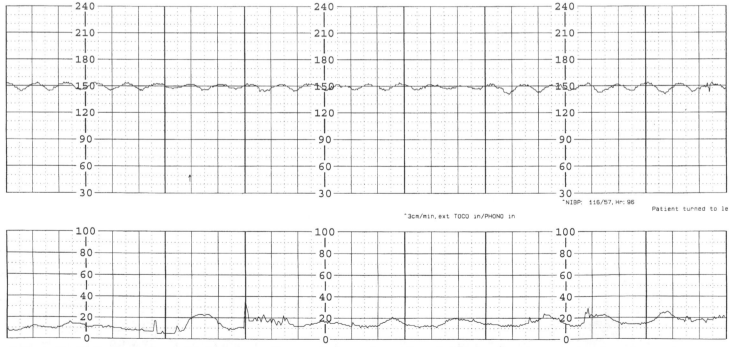

6.7   *Pathological sinusoidal pattern. Count the number of cycles in each minute.*

Did you see 2¹/2 cycles in the first minute, 2¹/2 cycles in the second minute, and 2 cycles in the third minute? Sinusoidal patterns or sinusoidal baselines have 1¹/2 to 5 cycles each minute. Pathologic sinusoidal patterns never have accelerations, but may have decelerations. Fetal movement is decreased or absent. Sometimes, a sinusoidal baseline waveform isn't symmetrical. The bottom portion of each cycle may dip lower than the upper portion of the cycle rises. But, it is still a sinusoidal pattern.

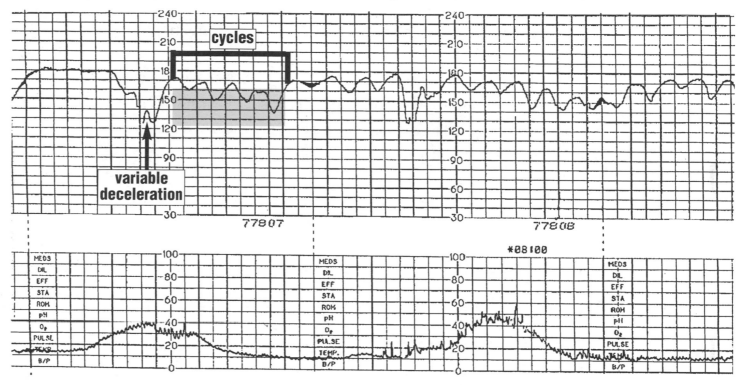

6.8   *Sinusoidal pattern with "V" shaped lower portion of cycles. Fetal hemoglobin was 6 gm/dl and the hematocrit was 18% at 33¹/2 weeks of gestation. Bleeding from placenta previa had occurred. Variable decelerations are also present.*

ACTIONS REQUIRED

When you see a sinusoidal pattern, it is important to
- assess fetal movement now and in the recent past

- review the entire tracing, there should be an acceleration within 100 minutes of monitoring

- assess maternal blood type. Rh negative? possibility of erythroblastosis fetalis?

- communicate your assessments to the midwife and/or physician
- act to increase fetal oxygenation.

BENIGN SINUSOIDAL PATTERN

Benign or physiologic sinusoidal patterns also have 1¹/2 to 5 cpm but decelerations are usually absent and accelerations are present before or after the sinusoidal baseline. Fetal movement may be present spontaneously or in response to acoustic or scalp stimulation. These patterns were called *pseudosinusoidal* in the past. These fetuses are not hypoxic, acidotic, or asphyxiated. They may be relaxed and making breathing, mouthing, or sucking movements, or simply reflecting the brainstem-cardiac response to narcotics.

To differentiate between a pathologic and a benign sinusoidal pattern:

*   obtain a fetal movement history

*   assess fetal movement by palpation, following acoustic stimulation, or real-time ultrasound

*   identify whether accelerations were present before the sinusoidal baseline began

*   identify the change in the FHR pattern after narcotic administration

*   relax! This is a benign pattern that requires no intervention.

Document this pattern's baseline rate, LTV, and acceleration(s). Most clinicians do not write "benign sinusoidal."

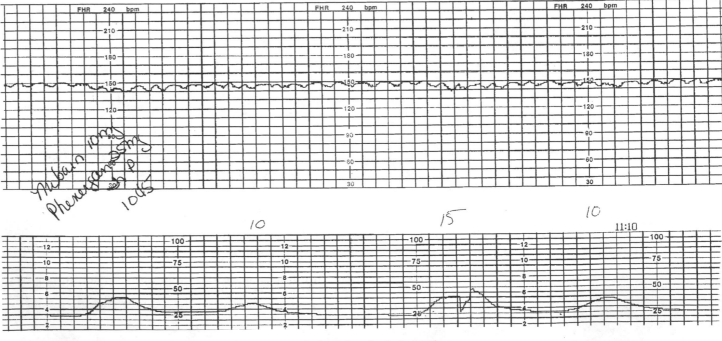

6.9   Benign sinusoidal pattern following Nubain® administration.

Essentials of Fetal Monitoring

Exercises

1. On the fetal monitor paper, draw 4 cycles per minute with average LTV. Show your drawing to a skilled clinician.

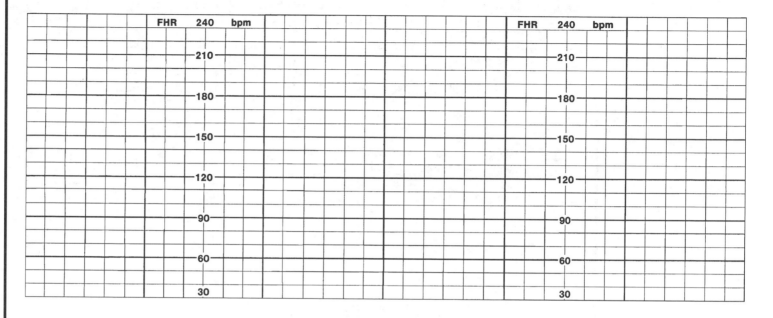

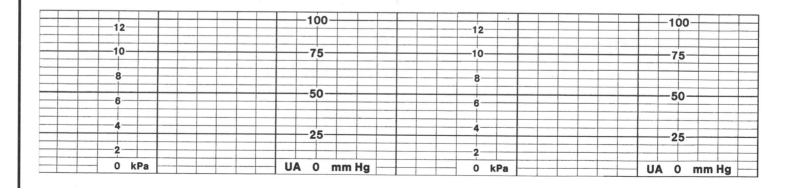

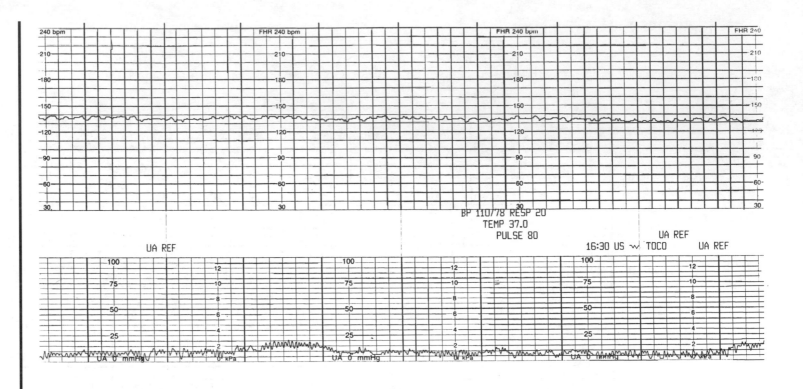

2. Classify LTV using a 5 category system.

   LTV is _____ to _____.

3. If there is only 1 cycle per minute, how would you classify LTV?

4. Match the type of LTV with its cause

   1. absent LTV   A. quiescent fetal state _____ (1 response)

   2. minimal LTV   B. narcotics _____ (2 responses)

   3. average LTV   C. compensation for an acute hypoxic event _____ (1 response)

   4. moderate LTV   D. neural integrity _____ (3 responses)

   5. marked LTV

5. LTV is categorized and recorded based on

    A. baseline bandwidth

    B. sine waves

    C. oscillations

    D. cycles per minute

6. A pathologic sinusoidal pattern can be obtained from a fetus with the following:

    A. narcotics "on board"

    B. hypoxia or acidosis

    C. sucking or mouthing

7. Which best describes categories for documentation of LTV?

    A. present or absent

    B. minimal, marked, moderate, increased, decreased

    C. absent, minimal, average, moderate, marked

    D. cpm, bpm

ANSWERS TO EXERCISES

1. show your instructor
2. minimal to average
3. absent LTV
4. A = 1, B = 1 & 2, C = 5, D = 2, 3, 4

5. A
6. B
7. C

SUMMARY

Summary

Long-term variability is a baseline characteristic with cycles and a bandwidth or amplitude. Cycles are also called sine waves, oscillations, or complexes. A special type of baseline is a sinusoidal baseline, also called a sinusoidal pattern. LTV can be classified using as many as 5 categories: absent, minimal, average, moderate, and marked. Depending on your facility, you may be asked to use less than 5 categories. The key question is, can you draw the baseline from your documentation description? Documenting more than one category, e.g., av to mod LTV, is acceptable because baselines fluctuate over time. **Absent and minimal LTV may be related to hypoxia. Marked LTV suggests fetal hypoxia**, usually from cord compression. Actions should be taken to improve fetal oxygenation. A return to average to moderate LTV with accelerations suggests interventions were successful.

SECTION 6:   LONG-TERM VARIABILITY

QUESTIONS

QUESTIONS

Directions: Circle T if the statement is true, F if it is false.

T	F	1.	Long-term variability has two components: sine waves and amplitude in beats per minutes.
T	F	2.	"Absent long-term variability" is documented if there are less than 1^1/2 cycles per minute.
T	F	3.	Persistent absent long-term variability with spontaneous accelerations and fetal movement suggests fetal asphyxia.
T	F	4.	A wandering baseline is the same as long-term variability.
T	F	5.	A pathologic sinusoidal pattern has long-term variability.
T	F	6.	To use long-term variability categories in documentation you must first identify the bandwidth of the baseline.
T	F	7.	Absent, minimal, and marked long-term variability require further assessments and possible actions to improve fetal oxygenation.
T	F	8.	Fetal sleep and awake cycles are accompanied by changes in long-term variability.
T	F	9.	"Present long-term variability" is clear terminology that enhances visualization of the tracing if the tracing is lost.
T	F	10.	Long-term variability is influenced by sympathetic and vagus nerves.

SECTION 7
Short-term Variability (STV)

Short-term variability is reflected on the fetal monitor's numeric display and paper by consecutive changes in the beats per minute (bpm) rate. Section 6 explained long-term variability cycles. Each cycle is the combination of consecutive printed rates. These consecutive rates might appear on the lighted display of the fetal monitor as 118, 119, 121, 118, 120, 122, 124, 121, etc. The changes from one bpm rate to the next bpm rate rarely exceed 8 bpm, e.g., 120 to 129 bpm. Usually the rates differ by 1 to 3 bpm. As each consecutive rate is printed on the moving fetal monitor paper, the baseline may appear bumpy, nonlinear, and/or chaotic. The bumpy look is called short-term variability. STV is a baseline characteristic. STV is not assessed in accelerations or decelerations. STV is usually documented as present or absent. Rarely, it is intermittent, with several minutes of STV and then several with absent STV.

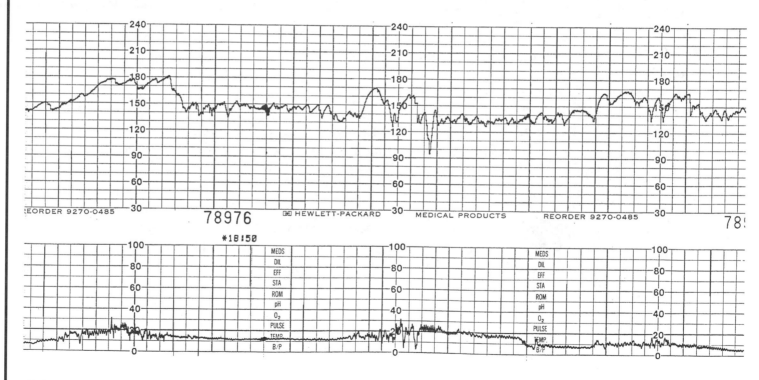

7.1 *STV is present, as are spontaneous accelerations to 162 to 180 bpm x 15-100 seconds. The baseline has a normal shift from 140-150 to 130-140 bpm. Long-term variability is average to moderate.*

**PHYSIOLOGY
OF STV**

**STV IS PRESENT
OR ABSENT**

**BEAT-TO-BEAT
VARIABILITY
(BTBV) IS
RELATED TO
SHORT-TERM
VARIABILITY
BUT IS NOT
SHORT-TERM
VARIABILITY**

Physiology of Short-term Variability

The vagus nerve is the 10th cranial nerve. It splits into two branches. The *right* vagal branch innervates the *sinoatrial (SA) node*. The *left* vagal branch innervates the *atrioventricular (AV) node*. The SA node is the heart's pacemaker, creating time fluctuations between heartbeats. **When the brainstem, vagus and SA node are oxygenated, STV will be present. When there is metabolic acidosis, asphyxia, or neurologic damage, STV will be absent**. Parasympatholytic drugs, such as scopolamine and atropine, decrease the differences between R to R (systole to systole) intervals and decrease STV. Narcotics may decrease LTV and STV.

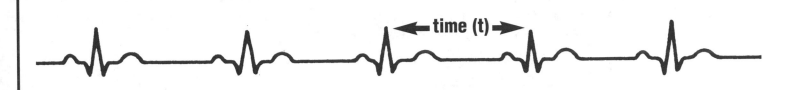

7.2   *If t= 0.5 seconds, the rate = 120 bpm. The beat-to-beat (time) interval will determine the bpm rate displayed and printed on the paper.* (Reproduced and modified with permission of Prentice-Hall, Inc. from Walraven, G. (1986). Basic Arrhythmias, p. 27).

The time interval between heartbeats, or systole, is measured 100% accurately when the fetal electrocardiogram (FECG) enters the fetal monitor via a spiral electrode in the fetus' buttocks or scalp. Changes in the R to R intervals change the calculated bpm rates and create STV. If the R to R intervals decrease, the bpm rate increases. When the R to R interval does not change, the baseline appears flat and smooth, like a rate calculated by a pacemaker. *The fluctuation in the time interval between consecutive heart beats is called beat-to-beat variability (BTBV).* BTBV is the interval between heartbeats and is not visible. BTBV is measured by the fetal monitor's computer in milliseconds (msec). **BTBV determines STV**. BTBV is determined by the fetal monitor's computer. STV is visible as a bumpy or rough appearance of the baseline. The presence of STV is reassuring. If BTBV is absent, STV will be absent. Absent STV may be nonreassuring and may require interventions to improve oxygenation if the absence of STV is not related to a central nervous system depressant drug.

DOCUMENTATION OF STV

The Association of Women's Health, Obstetric, and Neonatal Nurses (AWHONN) supports the use of a two-category system for charting STV, i.e., present or absent. Present STV is recorded as STV +. Absent STV is recorded as O STV, STV O, or STV –.

Look at the next two tracings.

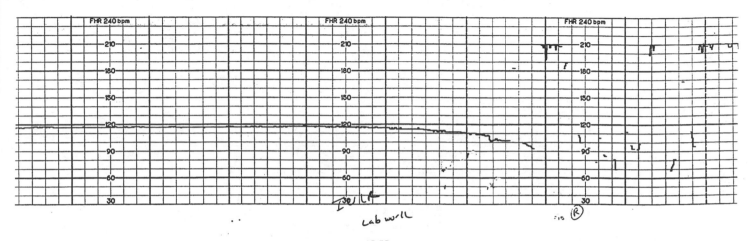

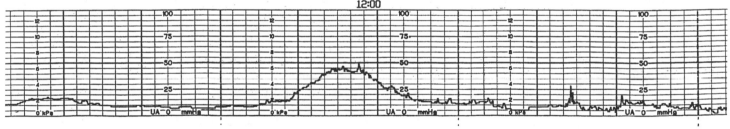

7.3   Short-term variability is absent.

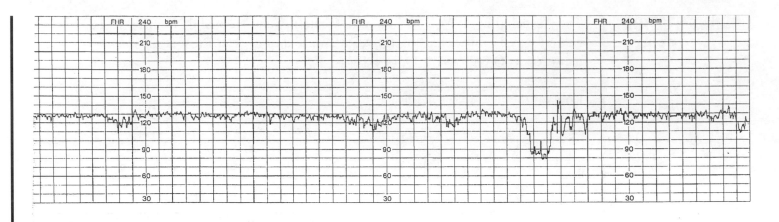

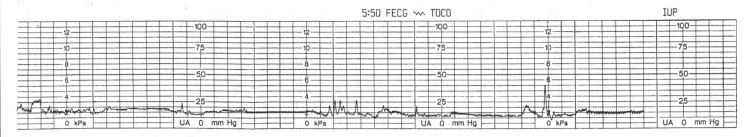

7.4   Short-term variability is present.

In the first tracing (7.3), STV is absent. In the second (7.4), STV is present. In both 7.3 and 7.4, LTV is absent as there are no visible cycles per minute in the baseline.

Exercises

Record STV for each tracing

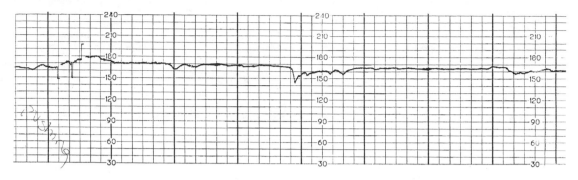

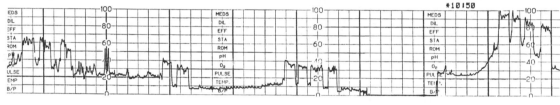

7.5   STV is _____

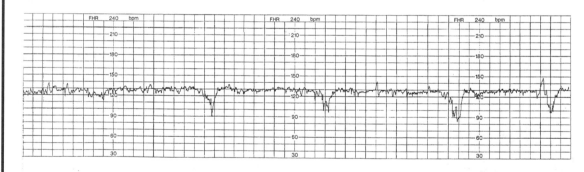

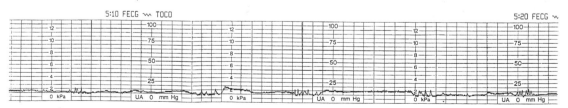

7.6   STV is _____

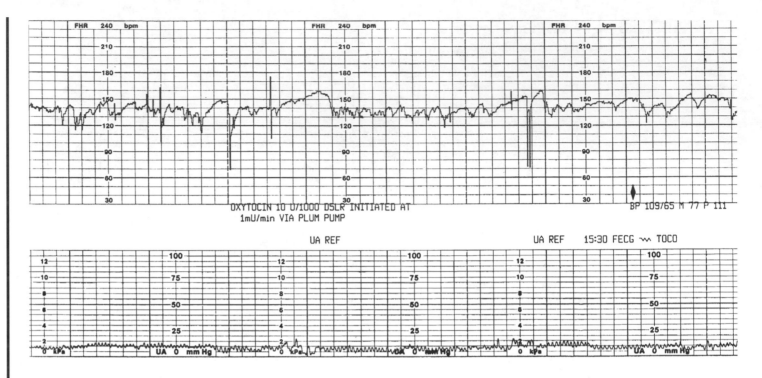

7.7   STV is _____

Did you say 7.5 STV is absent, 7.6 STV is present, and 7.7 STV is present? If you did, you're correct! When charting any aspect of the tracing, including STV, the assumption is that you viewed the tracing between the last time you charted and the current time you are charting. For example, the 1200 note might reflect your evaluation of the tracing since the 1145 note.

SIGNIFICANCE OF STV

Significance of STV

STV exists when there is an intact, oxygenated brainstem, parasympathetic nervous system, and heart conduction system. The vagus exerts a tonic effect and an oscillatory effect on the fetal heart rate (FHR). The tonic effect creates a drop in the baseline, decelerations, and bradycardia. Low voltage, fast electrocortical activity is associated with an increase in vagal tone, which would decrease the bpm change in STV. This happens when fetuses are in an "awake" state. So, while you may see accelerations in the FHR, STV will look small. Fetal vagal tone increases as gestation advances. Even preterm fetuses have STV.

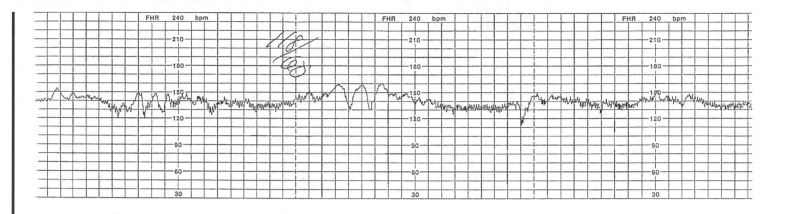

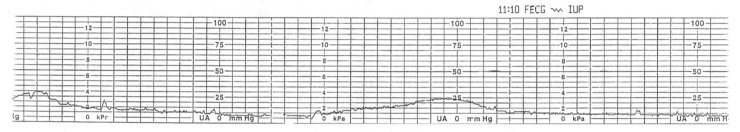

11:10 FECG ⌇ IUP

7.8 Accelerations with baseline short-term variability.

When STV is present:
- the vagus is intact and oxygenated and the brainstem, vagus, and heart are functioning.

STV:
- may fluctuate with fetal breathing movements (see 7.11)
- is influenced by baroreceptors, chemoreceptors, and catecholamines
- will increase or decrease due to fetal brain activity evidenced by changes in fetal "sleep/wake" states
- may be exaggerated in term and postterm **hypoxic** fetuses who release catecholamines (see 7.16)

STV decreases due to:
- parasympathetolytic drugs, such as atropine
- hypoxia, with the production of fetal adenosine and less SA nodal activity
- drugs, such as narcotics, which decrease neurologic function causing the **temporary** absence of STV

STV may be absent with:
- fetal sepsis, metabolic acidosis, asphyxia, brain death, or abnormal cardiac impulse conduction.

The Normal BPM Range of STV

Expect the lighted display on the fetal monitor to have bpm differences of 1 to 7 bpm between contractions and 4 to 8 bpm during contractions. STV bpm differences are rarely 9 to 10 bpm and **never** 15 or more bpm.

**STV IS
INCREASED
DURING
CONTRACTIONS**

Why would bpm differences increase during contractions rather than between contractions?

Contractions constrict maternal spiral arteries which diminishes blood flow to the placenta. This might cause a slight drop in oxygen delivery to the fetus and an increase in vagal tone. The actual cause of this increased STV is unknown.

**STV VS.
A DYSRHYTHMIA
SUCH AS PACS
OR PVCS**

When the fluctuation in consecutive FHRs is greater than 15 bpm, suspect premature atrial contractions (PACs) or premature ventricular contractions (PVCs). The following is an example of PACs. PACs are the most common fetal dysrhythmia.

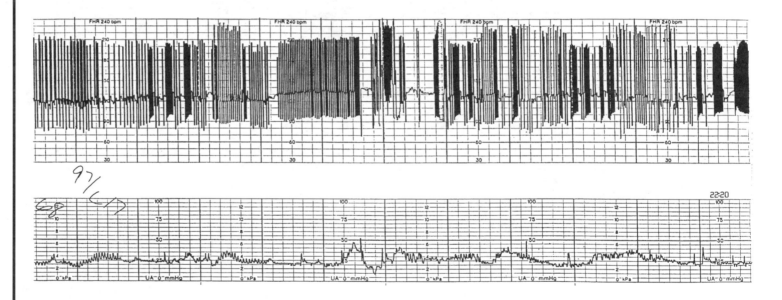

7.9   *Premature atrial contractions create the vertical line up and the compensatory pause creates an immediate line down. PACs are the most common fetal dysrhythmia.*

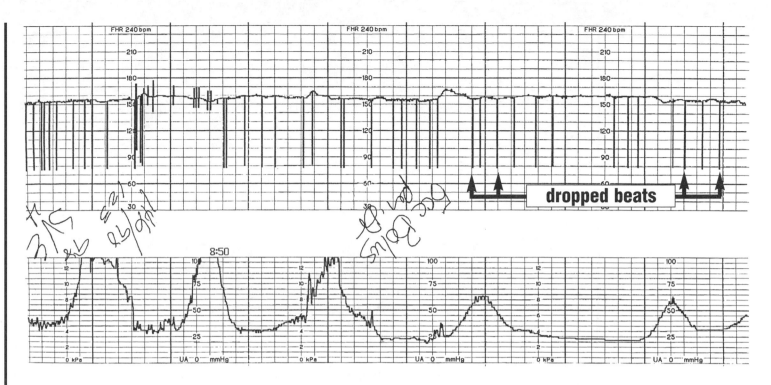

7.10 *Dropped beats due to a non-conducted sinoatrial (SA) node impulse. Note the baseline is near 160 bpm, and the bottom of the dropped beats is near 80 bpm (half the rate). These dropped beats reflect a 2 to 1 Mobitz II or second-degree heart block. The fetus is not acidemic (see the acceleration to 168 bpm x 25 seconds). An acceleration ≥ 10 bpm for ≥ 10 seconds rules out fetal acidemia.*

A dysrhythmia is not the same as STV. STV is the result of normal cardiac electrical conduction. PACs, PVCs, and heart block represent abnormal impulse conduction or a dysrhythmia. If you suspect PACs or PVCs, auscultate fetal heart tones with a fetoscope. An irregular rhythm suggests PACs or PVCs. Inform the midwife and/or physician. The pediatrician should also be informed as there is a small risk of a cardiac anomaly.

SAWTOOTH PATTERN

The Oscillatory Effect of the Vagus

The respiratory nerves and the nerves that regulate the vagus are next to each other in the brainstem. When the fetus inhales, the FHR may increase. With exhalation, the FHR may decrease. The result (a respiratory sinus dysrhythmia) is called a sawtooth pattern (7.11). A sawtooth pattern is rare, reassuring, and a sign of fetal well-being. Document "sawtooth pattern" and think of it as the same as STV is present.

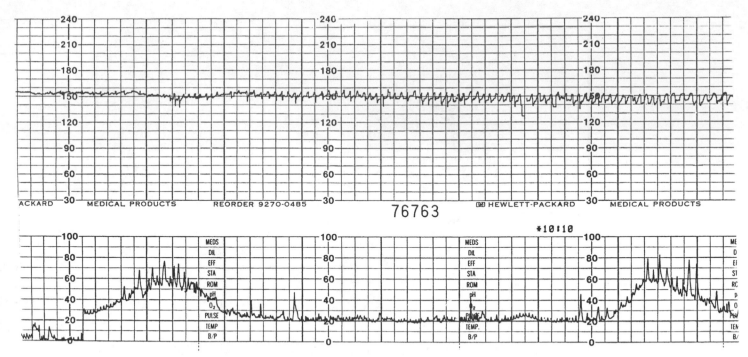

7.11   Sawtooth pattern due to the oscillatory effect of the vagus during fetal breathing movements.

The Ultrasound (US) and STV

US signal quality depends on placement of the transducer over the fetal heart, transducer pressure against the maternal abdomen, the quantity of adipose tissue (increasing the distance the US waves must travel), and the amount of coupling gel on the transducer face. If the US signal quality is good, and a fetal monitor with auto-correlation is used, the FHR will be calculated within 2.5 bpm of the true value. The printout will be similar to the printout generated when a spiral electrode is used. It has been said that the US record *very closely* approaches that of STV created when a spiral electrode is used. The tracing is a reasonable representation that is often *virtually identical* to the tracing printed when a spiral electrode is used. Sometimes, however, the US printout has less STV than the printout from a spiral electrode. **If it looks good on external, it probably is, but, there should be other evidence that the fetus is well, such as a reactive acceleration and fetal movement.**

STV has been documented by clinicians as present when the US is used, **but only when it's presence can be supported conceptually by the presence of a reactive acceleration**. A reactive acceleration peaks 15 or more bpm above the middle of the baseline and lasts 15 or more seconds at its base (7.12). If the US-generated tracing is flat with no accelerations, STV has been charted as absent. It is highly probable it is absent.

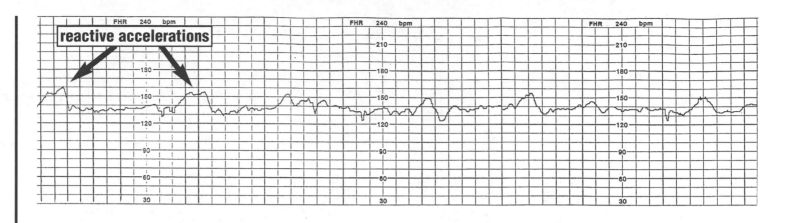

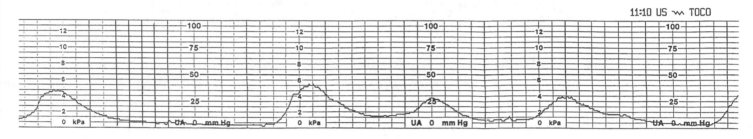

7.12 *An acceleration that peaks 15 or more bpm above the baseline and is 15 or more seconds at its base rules out metabolic acidosis. Short-term variability is conceptually present when the fetus is not acidotic, even with an ultrasound transducer in place. Therefore, it may be documented as present. However, many nurses hesitate to document STV until a spiral electrode is placed on the fetus.*

A REACTIVE
ACCELERATION
RULES OUT
METABOLIC
ACIDOSIS

THE ABSENCE OF
LTV AND NO
ACCELERATION
SUGGESTS STV
IS ABSENT

A reactive acceleration rules out metabolic acidosis. The presence of a reactive acceleration is reassuring. *STV is present when metabolic acidosis is absent* unless there is a congenital defect of the brain, heart, or autonomic nervous system that affects the vagus and prevents STV in spite of normal acid-base balance. Charting STV + is *conceptually correct* if the US-derived tracing has LTV and at least one reactive acceleration.

Another traditional saying is, **"If it looks bad on external, it's probably worse on internal."**

When the FHR baseline looks smooth on the US-derived tracing, you may document O STV, STV O, STV –, or STV absent. Metabolic acidosis or a dysrhythmia may cause a smooth tracing. Assess fetal movement. If it is present, a tachyarrhythmia is most likely present. The printer may be printing at half the actual rate. The fetal monitor is programmed to print up to the top of the paper scale. USA scale paper stops at 240 bpm. Therefore, any rate above 240 will print at half that rate (see 7.13).

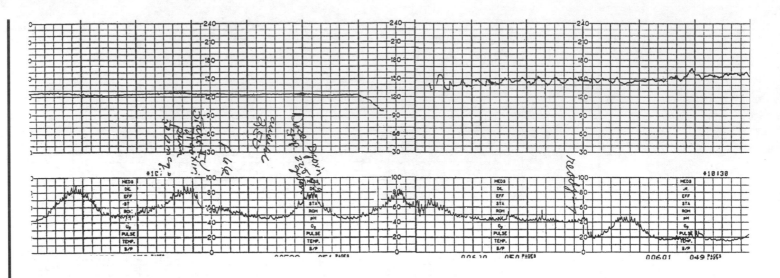

7.13 *The FHR due to fetal supraventricular tachycardia printed at half the actual rate before administration of maternal intravenous Digoxin. One and a half minutes after intravenous Digoxin, there was fetal cardioversion and the FHR returned to a normal rate.*

IF STV IS ABSENT, APPLY A SPIRAL ELECTRODE IF POSSIBLE

If STV is present and the fetus is not moving and has not moved for more than two hours, you may be monitoring the maternal heart rate. Confirm fetal life and the maternal heart rate. If STV is absent, and no central nervous system depressant drugs have been administered, assess maternal drug use. Notify the physician prior to the application of a spiral electrode to 100% accurately *measure* STV.

HEART BLOCK

STV is usually absent when congenital complete heart block (CCHB) or third degree heart block occurs (see 7.14). In this case, the fetus is usually active and well-oxygenated but SA nodal impulses are not transmitted to the atrioventricular (AV) node. The fetus with CCHB will decompensate when the FHR approaches 50 bpm and hydrops with congestive heart failure develops. Report this FHR to the physician as soon as possible. Try to stay calm. The fetus who is moving is not in any immediate danger. This is a dysrhythmia **not** a terminal bradycardia. A real-time ultrasound can be done to rule out hydrops and evaluate cardiac anatomy and the FHR. The woman will need to be transferred to the care of a perinatologist, and needs to be delivered where a pediatric surgeon is present during Cesarean section to place a temporary pacemaker in the newborn.

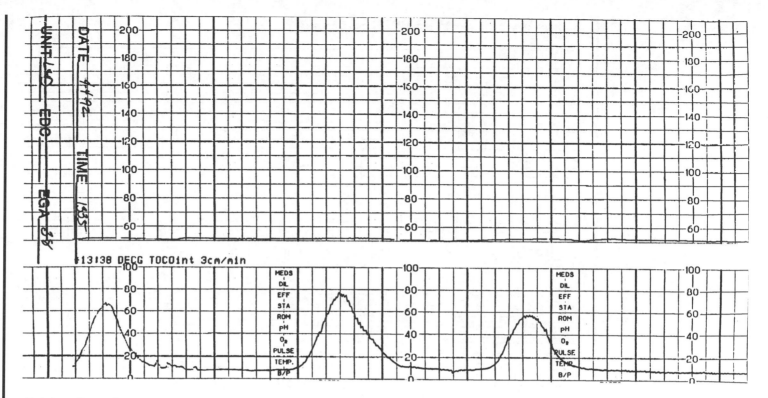

7.14   Complete heart block and European (International) scale paper.

The fetal heart rate is 51 to 53 bpm. The Apgars scores were 7 at 1 minute and 7 at 5 minutes, and mom was later diagnosed with lupus erythematosus. Half of all newborns with complete heart block have a mother with an antiphospholipid antibody syndrome such as lupus, Sjögren's syndrome, rheumatoid arthritis, Reynaud's syndrome or scleroderma. The other half of babies with CCHB have a congenital heart defect.

What Do You Do When STV is Absent?

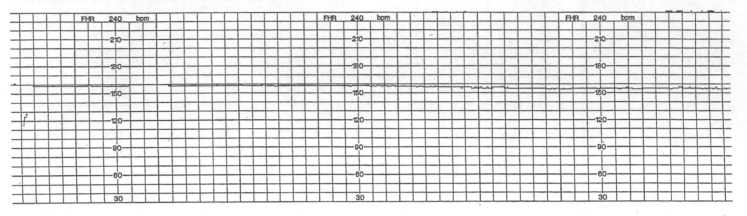

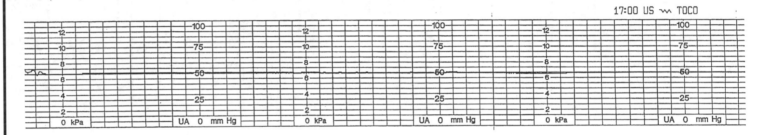

17:00 US ∿ TOCO

7.15   Absent STV. Absent LTV.

Actions in Response to Absent STV

- document O STV, STV O, STV-, absent STV, or STV absent

- obtain a maternal drug history and fetal movement history

- palpate fetal movement

- consider fetal hypoxia, anoxia, metabolic acidosis, and/or asphyxia

- perform a vaginal examination to determine the likelihood of a prompt vaginal delivery

- perform an ultrasound scan to assess fetal brain and heart anatomy and confirm the FHR

- take no actions if STV was present before a central nervous system depressant was given

- auscultate fetal heart tones with a fetoscope to confirm the rate. The FHR might be halving

- apply a spiral electrode to accurately measure STV.

If the baseline looks smooth (absent STV), and you suspect that the fetus needs oxygen, e.g., there has been a lack of fetal movement or accelerations for more than 100 minutes, enhance fetal oxygenation by increasing maternal cardiac output and blood oxygen content. To improve cardiac output and blood flow:

- change the mother's position so she is not supine, avoid Trendelenburg because it decreases cardiac output, avoid knee-chest (elbows and knees) when uterine rupture is suspected

- decrease uterine activity. Administer 500 or more ml of lactated Ringer's solution. To increase cardiac output, 1000 ml or more must be infused. Avoid this bolus if the woman is at increased risk for pulmonary edema, e.g., she is preeclamptic

- discontinue or remove oxytocic or prostaglandin agents (especially if uterine hyperstimulation occurs)

- give a tocolytic such as 0.25 mg terbutaline subcutaneously or intravenously if ordered by a physician or midwife (hold medication if abruption is suspected as this may worsen or mask the abruption).

Then, to improve blood oxygen content, apply a tight fitting simple face mask at 8 to 10 liters per minute of 100% oxygen or a partial rebreathing mask (with an oxygen reservoir bag) at 12 liters per minute. Oxygen should reach the fetus within 9 minutes. Is the FHR better by 10 minutes? Communicate your assessment and actions to the physician or midwife. Since the fetus should be out of a quiescent state by 100 minutes, look at the tracing to determine when the last acceleration occurred. Evaluate the fetal response. There is a saying when a fetus is metabolically acidotic: **"Once STV is gone, it's too late."**

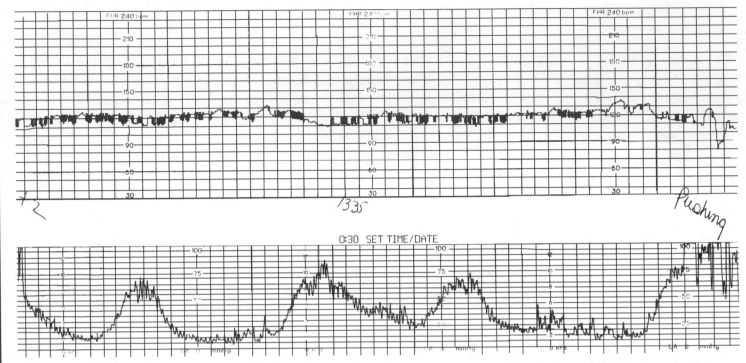

7.16   *Exaggerated STV may be due to fetal hypoxia. The presence of accelerations rule out metabolic acidosis. Hypoxia in this example may be due to uterine hyperstimulation.*

<table>
<tr><td>**EXAGGERATED
STV**</td><td>

Actions in Response to Exaggerated STV

Fetal hypoxia may stimulate the release of norepinephrine which affects sodium ions to increase the excitability of the SA node, increasing its oscillatory effect on the FHR, and exaggerating STV. Assess and record:

- exaggerated STV as STV + or STV present

- fetal heart tones with a fetoscope to rule out an irregular rhythm (dysrhythmia)

- maternal blood pressure to rule out hypo- or hypertension as a cause of hypoxia

- the last acceleration and fetal movement

- amniotic fluid color, amount, and odor

- actions to increase maternal uterine blood flow and oxygen delivery if hypoxia is suspected

- fetal response to your actions.

STV should return to a normal range after these actions.

</td></tr>
</table>

Summary

- BTBV is the fluctuation in pulse intervals between consecutive heartbeats. It is not visible, and it is measured by the fetal monitor in milliseconds. STV is measured in bpm

- BTBV determines STV

- STV is not assessed in accelerations or decelerations

- STV is a baseline characteristic

- STV is visualized on the FHR printout

- STV is documented as present or absent

- STV is chaotic, nonlinear, and may even look like small lines 9 to 10 bpm long

- a sawtooth pattern is similar to STV and reflects the FHR when there is a respiratory sinus dysrhythmia

- the baseline appears smooth when pulse intervals are similar

- the presence of STV is a sign of fetal well-being and brainstem oxygenation. If decelerations exist, intervene in response to the decelerations

- the absence of STV suggests possible metabolic acidosis, CNS depression from a drug such as a tranquilizer, narcotic, nicotine, magnesium sulfate, or fetal quiet sleep, anencephaly, injury to the brainstem, a dying fetus, brain death, infection, trauma, or cardiovascular defects

- when STV is absent, the digital readout will not change or will not be greater than 1 bpm between calculated rates and the baseline will be smooth

- determine the most likely reason for absent STV, intervene accordingly, and communicate your assessments and actions.

Exercises

1. What is the bpm (STV) range expected between contractions? _____ to _____ bpm

2. What is the bpm range expected during contractions? _____ to _____ bpm

3. Document STV as present or absent.

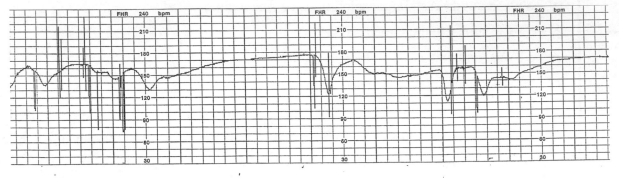

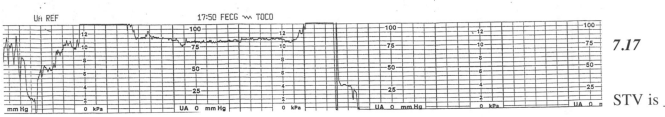

7.17

STV is _____

4.   Document STV as present or absent.

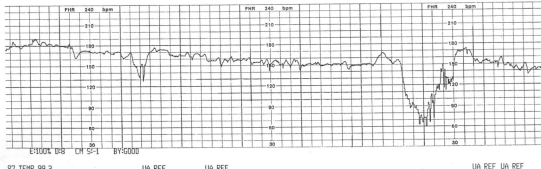

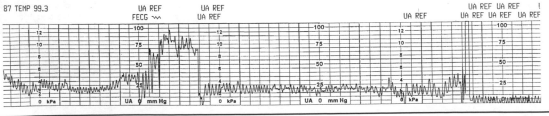

7.18

STV is _____

1. 1-7
2. 4-8
3. absent
4. present

SECTION 7:   SHORT-TERM VARIABILITY

QUESTIONS

QUESTIONS

Directions: Circle T if the statement is true, F if it is false.

T   F   1.   Beat-to-beat variability is measured in beats per minute.

T   F   2.   The presence of a reactive acceleration strongly suggests short-term variability is present.

T   F   3.   A sawtooth pattern is a sign of central nervous system compromise.

T   F   4.   When STV is exaggerated, the fetus may be hypoxic.

T   F   5.   The absence of STV is always synonymous with metabolic acidosis.

T   F   6.   STV can be 100% accurately *measured* when a spiral electrode is on the fetus.

T   F   7.   STV is a deceleration characteristic.

T   F   8.   Even if the fetus has complete heart block, short-term variability will be present.

T   F   9.   Supplemental oxygen should reach the fetus by 9 or fewer minutes.

T   F   10.   When short-term variability is present, it is never necessary to intervene.

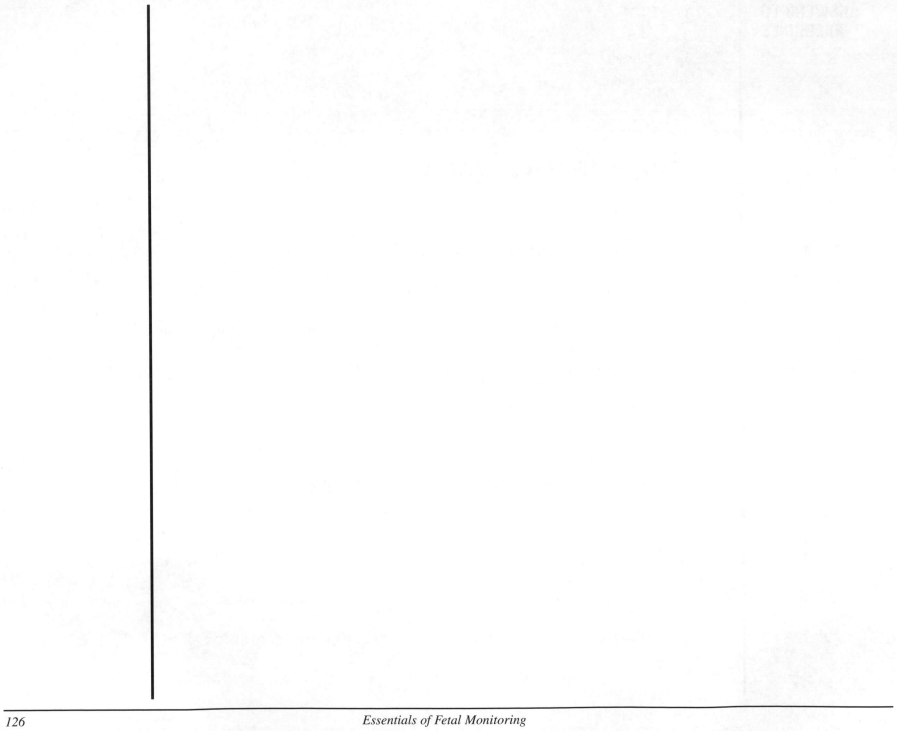

Essentials of Fetal Monitoring

SECTION 8
Accelerations (Accels)

Variability and accelerations are two separate concepts. Accelerations are a transient increase in the fetal heart rate (FHR) above the baseline. They may be as small as a 10 bpm increase lasting 10 or more seconds. If the acceleration peaks at least 15 beats per minute (bpm) above the baseline and lasts 15 or more seconds at its base, it is called a **reactive** acceleration.

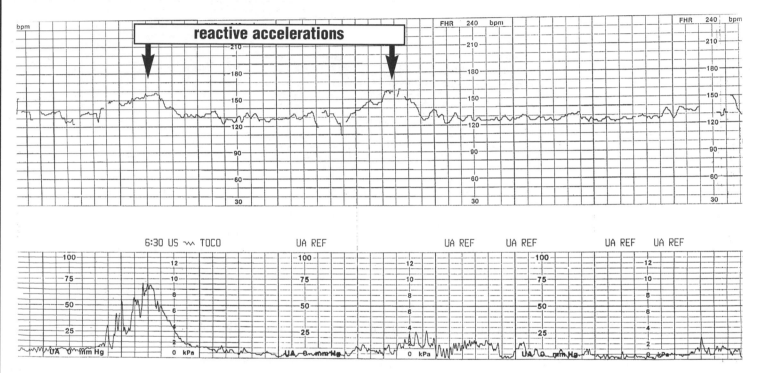

8.1   *The baseline is 122 to 134 bpm with spontaneous accelerations to 160 x 60-65 seconds. This is a reassuring pattern.*

The rise above the baseline and the duration of accelerations can be measured. To determine the amplitude or height of the acceleration, the average baseline rate is first identified. Estimate the bpm increase to the acceleration peak. The duration is measured from the beginning of the onset of the acceleration until it returns to the baseline. Spontaneous accels vary in shape from one to the next. Therefore, the height and duration might be charted using a range, e.g., accels to 160-165 bpm x 55-60 seconds.

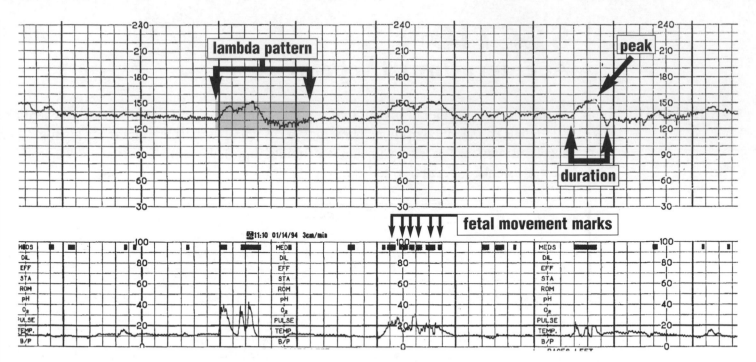

8.2   ***These spontaneous accelerations peak at 150 to 152 bpm and have a duration of 25-65 seconds. The FHR dips slightly after the first acceleration. This is a normal response and is due to a baroreceptor stimulus and vagal response following the increase in the FHR and BP during the acceleration. An accelertion with a "dip" is called a Lambda pattern and is innocuous. Note the fetal movement marks at the top of the uterine activity channel. This was created by a Hewlett-Packard® monitor.***

SPONTANEOUS ACCELS

Spontaneous accels usually increase by 10 bpm or more above the BL. They are an obvious "bump" that could stand alone. They vary in shape from one to the next but occasionally look similar as they can all have a pointed peak. They usually are at their peak in less than 20 seconds.

REACTIVE ACCELS

Reactive accels are defined by their size. They increase at least 15 bpm and last at least 15 seconds. One reactive acceleration rules out metabolic acidosis.

A *reactive* nonstress test (NST) exists when there are at least two reactive accelerations that peak 15 bpm above the baseline and last 15 seconds at their base in a 20 minute tracing. Most people use the middle of the baseline to begin their measurement to the peak of the acceleration. If a NST is not reactive by 40 minutes, the physician should be notified so that additional tests may be ordered. All fetuses should accelerate by the 100th minute of monitoring.

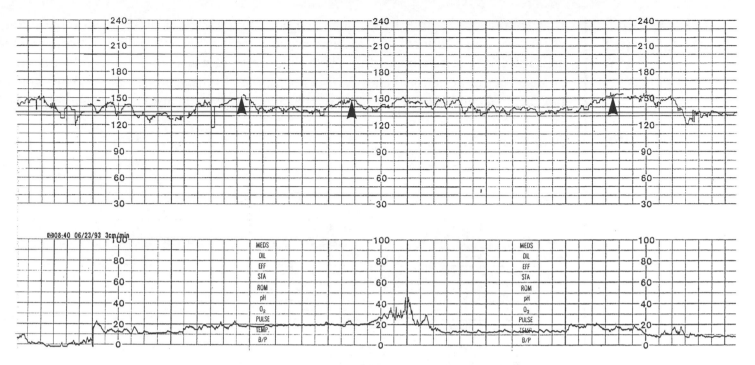

8.3   Select the middle of the baseline prior to measuring acceleration height or amplitude.

Reactivity has been used in some medical articles to mean reactive. However, since there is confusion as to the meaning of reactivity (some think it means variability is "good"), it is best **not** to use this word in communication and documentation.

Prematurity and Accelerations

*   accels begin at 15 to 16 weeks of gestation

*   the neurologic system is thought to be mature after 30 weeks of gestation. After 30 weeks, you should expect to see many "15 x 15" accels

*   prior to 32 weeks of gestation expect to see many "10 x 10" accels but also some "15 x 15" accels

*   "15 x 15" reactive accels are present in 16.7% of fetuses who are 23-27 weeks of gestation

*   "15 x 15" reactive accels are present in 65.6% of fetuses who are 28-32 weeks of gestation

*   "15 x 15" reactive accels are present in 90.6% of fetuses who are 33-37 weeks of gestation

Accelerations (10 bpm x 10 seconds) in a preterm fetus less than 32 weeks of gestation are **not** documented as reactive for gestational age. More research is needed to confirm the relationship between "10 x 10" accels and the lack of metabolic acidosis. Usually prior to 32 weeks of gestation, the tracing is interpreted as "FHR appropriate for gestational age" or "not appropriate for gestational age." A fetus who accelerates is most likely **not** metabolically acidotic. However, a reactive acceleration always rules out metabolic acidosis.

Exercise

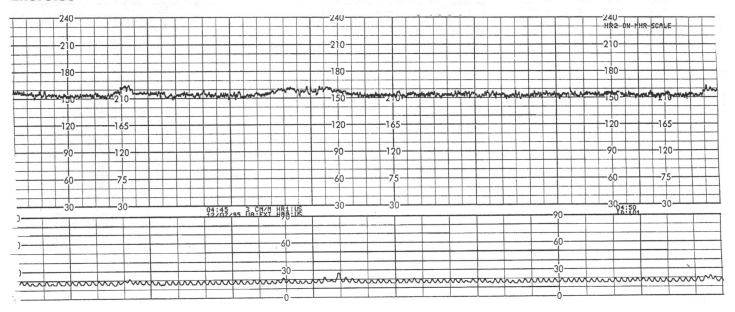

8.4   Baseline 150-154 bpm with accelerations to 162 bpm x 15-50 seconds. The maternal hemoglobin was 6.5 gm/dl. The fetus was most likely not metabolically acidotic but may have been hypoxic.

Look at this tracing (8.4). Is it reactive? If you said no, you are correct. The accelerations did not meet strict "15 x 15" criteria. This does not mean the fetus is acidotic, it just means the accelerations weren't big enough to call the tracing reactive. Preterm fetuses begin to accelerate their FHR at 15 to 16 weeks of gestation. As the fetus matures, higher and longer accelerations occur. Research has shown that a "15 x 15" accel rules out metabolic acidosis and a "10 x 10" acceleration rules out acidemia. More research is needed to determine if smaller accelerations also rule out metabolic acidosis.

ANTENATAL ACCELS

Accels present in an NST have a greater than 99% negative predictive value. That means a reactive NST predicts fetal well-being in 99 of 100 babies at the time of the NST. The frequency and number of NSTs is based on maternal/fetal risk factors.

SPONTANEOUS AND UNIFORM ACCELS

There are two kinds of accelerations: spontaneous accels and uniform accels. They can occur any time, i.e., between or during contractions. The fetal physiologic response prior to each type of acceleration is different. Spontaneous accelerations may be preceded by a sensory stimulus such as scalp pH sampling, scalp stimulation, or acoustic stimulus. Uniform accelerations are preceded by mild cord compression where the umbilical vein is compressed but the arteries are not. The drop in fetal pO_2 and blood pressure triggers chemoreceptors and baroreceptors. A message travels to the brainstem via Hering's nerves and the glossopharyngeal nerves. Sympathetic nerves are stimulated, and the fetal heart rate increases.

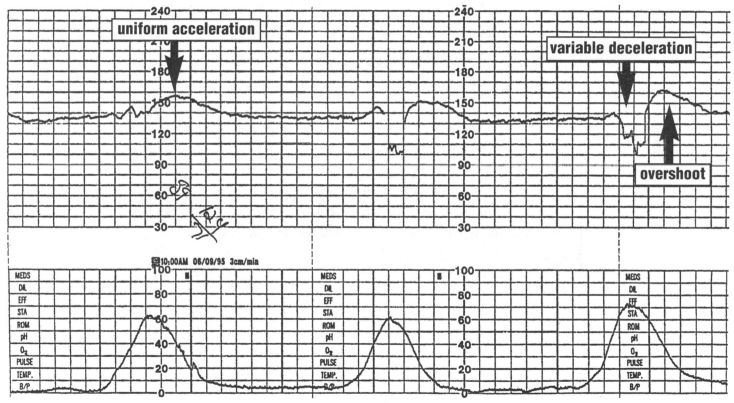

8.5 *Uniform accelerations reflect mild cord compression. Could there be oligohydramnios? The overshoots represent fetal catecholamine release.*

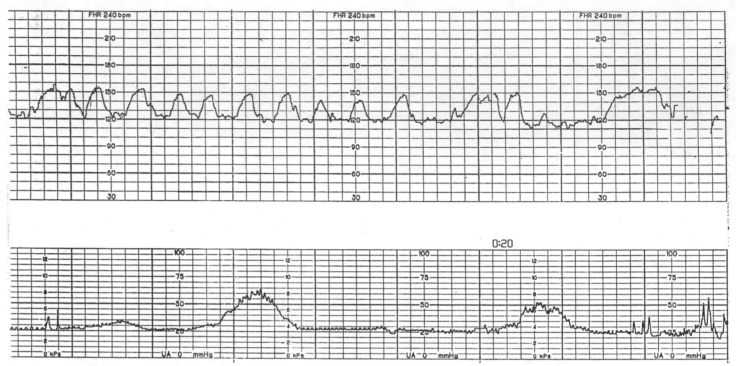

8.6 *Fetus in an active awake (4F) state with multiple spontaneous accelerations and a baseline near 120 bpm.*

LABOR ACCELS

Accelerations During Labor

A reactive, spontaneous accel indicates the absence of a metabolically acidotic fetus at the time of the acceleration. A reactive uniform accel is also indicative of a nonacidotic fetus, but oligohydramnios may exist. Oligohydramnios is a chronic hypoxia marker in an anatomically normal fetus.

Expect spontaneous accels during labor. Well fetuses move during labor 30 to 40 times an hour and should accelerate each and every hour. If concern exists about fetal well-being, a spiral electrode (SE) should be applied to accurately measure short-term variability. If the cervix is not dilated enough to insert the SE or if there is a contraindication to rupture of the membranes, a real-time ultrasound may be needed to assess fetal movement, fetal breathing, fetal anatomy, amniotic fluid volume, and to demonstrate fetal well-being. No woman should leave your facility until fetal well-being is firmly established, even if the woman is not in labor or is in false or early labor. Remember to respond to fetal physiology. If the vertex is accessible, scalp rubbing, known as scalp stimulation, can be used to create a sensory nerve/sympathetic nerve stimulus and an acceleration to rule out metabolic acidosis.

To distinguish spontaneous accels from uniform accels, compare their shapes. Uniform accels reach their peak in 20 or more seconds, have a slanted onset, and are often round (like a hump on a camel's back). Spontaneous accels peak in less than 20 seconds. Upside down, spontaneous accelerations look like variable decelerations but uniform accels look like late decelerations.

PROLONGED ACCELS

Prolonged accels may be confused with tachycardia when the FHR stays above 160 bpm for 2 or more minutes. Fetuses with a prolonged accel should be actively moving. Abdominal palpation confirms fetal movement. Some fetuses can stay in the active awake state up to two hours which delays baseline identification. As long as there are no decelerations, prolonged accelerations strongly suggest an uncompromised, well-oxygenated fetus.

SUMMARY

Summary

Accelerations are transient, obvious increases in the FHR above the baseline. A reactive nonstress test (NST) has at least two accelerations in a 20 minute period and each acceleration peaks 15 or more bpm above the baseline and lasts 15 or more seconds at its base. To determine accel height or amplitude, use the average baseline rate then measure 15 bpm above it. A reactive NST predicts a well-oxygenated fetus at the time of the test. NSTs are usually called reactive or nonreactive at 32 or more weeks of gestation. Prior to 32 weeks, the test is usually interpreted as FHR "appropriate for gestational age" or "not appropriate for gestational age." An NST is analyzed after 40 minutes of monitoring or less. The physician should be notified if it is nonreactive. All fetuses should accelerate by the end of 100 minutes of monitoring. If a spiral electrode cannot be applied or scalp stimulation cannot be done to determine fetal well-being, acoustic stimulation or a real-time ultrasound should be done to assess fetal movement and/or to elicit accelerations.

"Reactivity" is poorly defined in the literature and should not be used in communication or documentation. The presence of accelerations that do not meet "reactive" criteria still suggests a nonacidotic fetus. More research is needed to confirm that smaller accelerations also rule out metabolic acidosis. Fetuses can accelerate for two or more minutes when they are in an active awake state. The presence of fetal movement and the absense of decelerations suggests fetal well-being. Uniform accelerations reflect mild umbilical cord compression that may be due to cord vulnerability and oligohydramnios. If uniform accelerations appear during an antepartal test, an ultrasound to determine cord position and fluid volume may reveal oligohydramnios.

Accelerations (Accels)

SECTION 8: ACCELERATIONS

QUESTIONS

QUESTIONS

Directions: Circle T if the statement is true, F if it is false.

T F 1. Nonstress tests are reactive if they have two "10 x 15" accelerations in a 20 minute period.

T F 2. It is not an acceleration unless it is 15 beats above baseline and lasts 15 seconds at its base.

T F 3. Acceleration height for a nonstress test is usually measured from the bottom of the baseline.

T F 4. Accelerations are related to fetal acid-base status.

T F 5. Reactive accelerations must be sustained at the top for 15 or more seconds.

T F 6. By 33 weeks of gestation, 90% of fetuses have reactive accelerations.

T F 7. If one acceleration lasts 2 minutes, you can classify the tracing as reactive.

T F 8. If two "10 x 15" accelerations are present in 20 minutes and the fetus is 26 weeks of gestation, the NST is not appropriate for gestational age.

T F 9. More than half of fetuses less than 27 weeks of gestation have "15 x 15" accelerations.

T F 10. "Reactive for gestational age" is acceptable language to document the NST result of a preterm fetus.

SECTION 9
Early Decelerations (Early decels)

PERIODIC DECELERATIONS

Early Decelerations are Periodic in Timing

Decelerations that occur in response to pressure exerted during contractions are called periodic decelerations. The three types of periodic decelerations are early, late, and variable decelerations. Variable decelerations can also occur between contractions.

PERIODIC DECELERATIONS/WITH CONTRACTIONS	
Pressure is on the	Type of Deceleration
• **fetal head**	• **early**
• uterine vessels	• late
• umbilical cord	• variable

PHYSIOLOGY OF EARLY DECELERATIONS

Early decelerations are rare. They occur in approximately 3% of all labors and **never** occur prior to labor. They reflect a vagal response as a result of *increased* intracranial pressure and *decreased* blood flow through blood vessels in the brain. There may also be a constriction of the carotid arteries preceding the vagal slowing of the fetal heart rate (FHR). When early decels occur, the baby's body is usually well-oxygenated but the brain is compressed more than normal. Expect to see accelerations and short-term variability as a sign of fetal well-being. Persistent abnormally strong head compressions could result in a cephalohematoma or a brain bleed such as a subdural hemorrhage. In rare cases, the brain hemorrhage may cause brain damage and cerebral palsy. Early decelerations do not increase our concern for fetal hypoxia. They increase our concern for brain trauma.

4 TO 7 CM

Early decelerations are usually apparent when the cervix presses on the anterior fontanel between 4 to 7 centimeters of dilatation. Therefore, early decelerations will not exist between 0 and 4 cm. You will never see early decelerations during an antepartal test such as a nonstress test. Early decelerations may occur between 7 and 10 cm if enough force is exerted on the fetal head to cause a vagal response. However, at and after 10 cm of dilatation, the vagal response from head and cord compression usually produces sharp drops in the FHR, or variable decelerations.

CAPUT

Caput or caput succedaneum is scalp edema due to subcutaneous serum collection and fluid accumulation. Pressure on the scalp from the cervix obstructs venous return and creates caput. Caput only occurs *after* rupture of the membranes. Increasing caput indicates the need to reassess the labor situation to rule out CPD. Caput crosses the sutures. It is indentable. Caput usually resolves 24 to 36 hours after birth.

MOLDING

Molding is the ability of the fetal head to change shape to fit the maternal pelvis. Ideally, molding occurs slowly so no brain damage occurs. Excessive molding can cause extreme compression and can potentially cause brain damage from hemorrhage. Therefore, molding is a greater concern than caput. Molding is determined by palpating overriding skull bones (overlapping bony plates of the skull) and noting that the fontanels may be compressed and feel smaller than anticipated.

CPD RISK BUT NOT HYPOXIA

Fetuses who have caput and molding are adapting the shape of their head to the maternal pelvis and have an increased risk of cephalopelvic disproportion (CPD). Document and communicate caput and/or molding to the certified nurse midwife and/or physician. Early decelerations can be associated with CPD. Monitor fetal descent. The lack of descent may be associated with CPD, especially if the vertex is higher than the ischial spines.

REASSURING PATTERN, EMOTIONALLY CONCERNED

Caput and molding can occur with a tight head-to-pelvis fit. Even though early decelerations are part of a reassuring (nonhypoxic) FHR pattern (accelerations should exist too), nurses, midwives, and physicians should still be concerned about the risk of CPD. Will the baby fit? Is a vaginal route of delivery probable or improbable? What signs of fetal well-being are still in evidence?

CAPUT, MOLDING, CERVICAL EDEMA, AND LABOR PROGRESS

Possible Actions in Response to Early Decelerations

Early decelerations should be reported to the midwife and/or physician. In addition, the clinician may:
- plot a labor curve (see Section 4)
  - is progress delayed?
- assess the cervix
  - 4 to 7 cm?
  - swollen?
- assess station and the fetal head
  - caput?
  - molding?

Recognition Criteria

Early decels begin 10 to 20 seconds after the contraction begins, their lowest point or nadir is less than 18 seconds after the peak of the contraction. Therefore, **the nadir lag time for early decels is < 18 seconds**. Early decels have a slanted onset and offset, and a saucer or bowl shape. Early decels are back to the baseline close to the end of the contraction (see 9.1). To reiterate, the contraction peak to decel nadir duration is known as lag time. The lag time for early decels is < 18 seconds. Early decels are similar in shape.

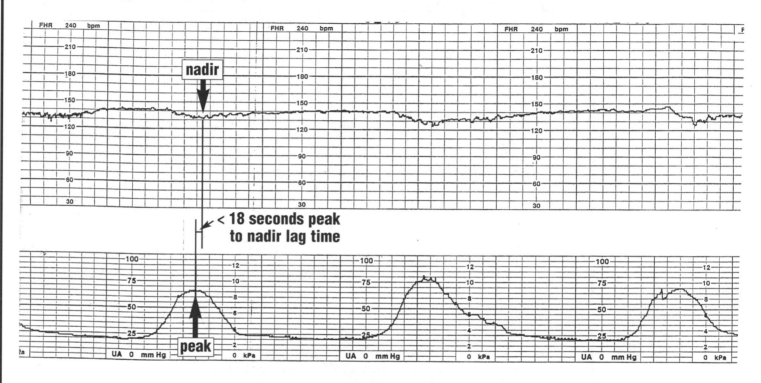

9.1   *The baseline is 140-143 bpm. Early decelerations are present but long-term variability is absent. Note the nadir (lowest point) of the deceleration occurs within 18 seconds after the contraction peak.*

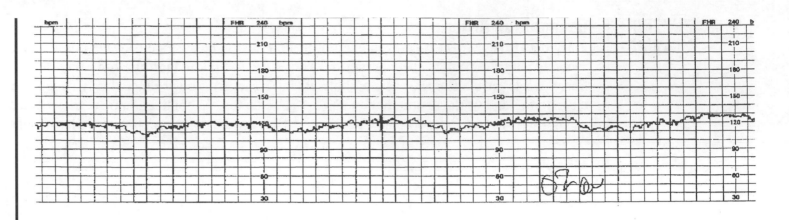

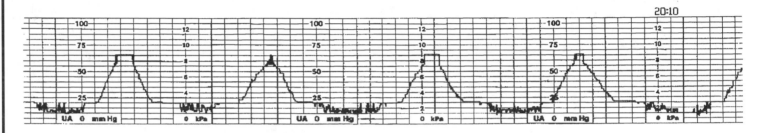

9.2 *The baseline is 118-120 bpm and 120-125 bpm. Short-term variability and early decelerations are present. Was oxygen needed? Note the contraction peak to deceleration nadir lag time is less than 18 seconds.*

DOCUMENTATION

Document "early decels." Since early decelerations represent head compression, their duration and depth are not clinically significant. Therefore, there is no need to document duration and depth. Oxygen is not needed since the fetus is not hypoxic. Be sure to document signs of fetal well-being such as fetal movement, accelerations, and short-term variability.

Review the prenatal record. What is the woman's height and weight gain? Could there be CPD? Estimate fetal weight. Measure fundal height. Does it seem high for gestational age?

Plot a labor curve. Is descent delayed? If so, there may be CPD.

Document your findings regarding dilatation, effacement, station, caput, and molding. Notify the midwife or physician of caput and/or molding and of any concerns you have regarding fetal fit. For example, "Early decels. 5' 3", 185 lbs., EFW (estimated fetal weight) 8 lbs., 5/90%/0 with caput, no molding. Midwife notified of early decels and SVE (sterile vaginal examination) findings. No further orders at this time. Plan is to continue observation of dilatation and descent."

WHEN EARLY DECELS ARE DOCUMENTED BUT THE HEAD IS NOT COMPRESSED

What if, after performing an SVE, you decide the fetal head is high and not compressed? Or, what if the woman is dilated only 2 to 3 cm? Then the most likely cause of the vagal response or deceleration was cord compression. If "early decels" was charted, don't change your entry. We document the picture we see then confirm with our actions. A logical assumption is the cord is compressed. Try a position change to see which position results in smaller decelerations. Then look for short-term variability. Palpate fetal movement and note any accelerations (all signs of fetal well-being). Document these signs of fetal well-being, i.e., fetal movement, accelerations, and short-term variability.

SUMMARY

Summary

Early decelerations are caused by a vagal response following increased intracranial pressure. They usually occur during contractions between 4 to 7 cm of dilatation. They are associated with CPD and as long as there are accelerations, fetal movement, and STV, the pattern is reassuring and reflective of a nonacidotic fetus. Be concerned about CPD, arrested labor progress, caput, and molding. If the head is not compressed, the vagal response and deceleration is most likely caused by umbilical cord compression.

SECTION 9: EARLY DECELERATIONS

QUESTIONS

Directions: Circle T if the statement is true, F if it is false.

QUESTIONS

T   F

T   F

T   F

T   F

T   F

T   F

T   F

T   F

T   F

T   F

1.   Early decelerations occur during the antepartal period.

2.   Early decelerations often occur when the cervix is dilated 1-3 cm.

3.   Early decelerations are associated with cephalopelvic disproportion.

4.   Caput can occur before rupture of the membranes.

5.   It is important to document the depth and duration of early decelerations.

6.   If the fetal head is not compressed but the decelerations meet all the criteria of early decelerations, the next most likely cause of the decelerations is cord compression.

7.   Early decelerations result from decreased intracranial pressure and increased blood flow through the cerebral blood vessels.

8.   Early decelerations may be the result of pressure on the posterior fontanel.

9.   Early decelerations are a precursor of possible brain trauma.

10.   Early decelerations only occur when there is caput and molding.

SECTION 10
Late and Spontaneous Decelerations

PERIODIC DECELERATIONS/WITH CONTRACTIONS	
Pressure is on the	Type of Deceleration
• fetal head	• early
• **uterine vessels**	• **late**
• umbilical cord	• variable

A late deceleration reflects fetal hypoxia caused by diminished blood flow through uterine or placental vessels. This diminished blood flow is called uteroplacental insufficiency. Late decelerations are periodic in their timing, i.e., they only occur in response to contractions which squeeze maternal spiral arteries (arteries in the uterus) and decrease oxygen to the placenta. Late decelerations may also be a response to placental abruption or maternal hypotension. There can be just one late deceleration, an intermittent appearance of a late deceleration, or repetitive late decelerations. Five or more late decelerations in a row is called a pattern of late decelerations.

Recognition Criteria

RECOGNITION CRITERIA

Late decelerations are usually similar in shape from one to the next. Some are curved, some are shaped like a U or V, and some may appear "boxy." Late decelerations last up to 2 minutes. A deceleration that lasts longer than 2 minutes is called a prolonged deceleration. Prolonged decelerations are discussed in Section 12. You do **not** need internal monitors to determine if a late deceleration exists. You just need to recognize them and document them as late decelerations.

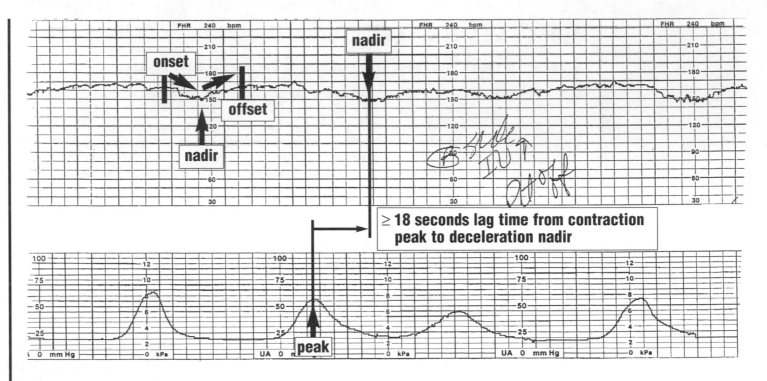

10.1 *Late decelerations. The nurse responded appropriately by turning the woman to her right side, increasing the intravenous fluid flow rate, and discontinuing Pitocin®.*

A late deceleration has a slanted, gradual onset but may have an abrupt recovery or offset. **Late decelerations begin after the contraction begins. The lowest point of the deceleration or nadir is always ≥ 18 seconds after the contraction peak.** When a tocotransducer is used to assess contractions, the uterine activity waveform may last longer than the actual contraction. As a result, the late deceleration may appear to return to the baseline (BL) before the contraction ends, even though all late decelerations return to the baseline after the contraction ends. Don't ignore or discount that late deceleration. The woman was probably tightening her abdominal muscles, increasing pressure on the tocotransducer (TOCO). Palpate the uterus. Document on the tracing the actual end of the contraction if you can. Also document in your notes "late decel" or "late decels" if more than one was seen. Document your actions in response to the late decels.

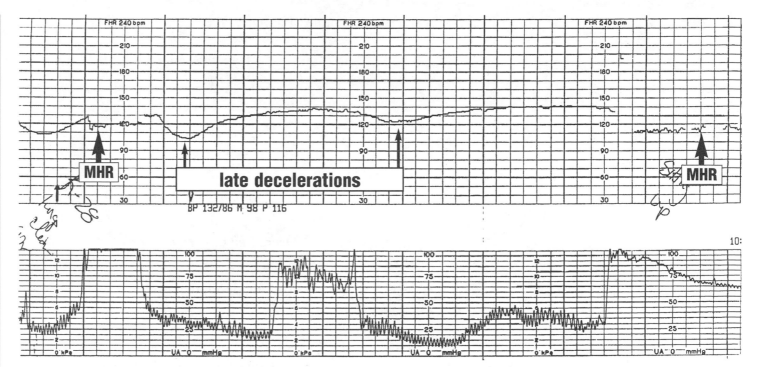

10.2 *During pushing with the first contraction, the maternal heart rate (MHR) of approximately 120 bpm is recorded. It is also recorded in the last minute of the strip. These late decelerations reach their nadir in 20-25 seconds. The nadir is ≥ 18 seconds after the contraction peak. The late decelerations are back to baseline after the contraction ends and are similar in shape.*

PHYSIOLOGY

During a contraction, especially those stronger than 35 mm Hg, oxygen delivery to the fetus is significantly curtailed. Well-oxygenated fetuses maintain a normal FHR during and after contractions. When a fetus has a borderline oxygen level, a late deceleration may appear. Inadequate oxygen delivery to the fetus is called *uteroplacental insufficiency*. **The fetus is hypoxic.** The presence of a reactive acceleration does not rule out a late deceleration but demonstrates the fetus is hypoxic but not yet metabolically acidotic.

The lack of oxygen may originate from maternal causes such as hypotension or uterine hyperstimulation and/or hypertonus, or placental causes such as villous edema, avascular villi, or placental calcifications or infarcts which can occur in women who smoke or who have diseases such as anticardiolipin antibody syndrome or lupus erythematosus. If hypoxia persists, eventually there will be the loss of accelerations and short-term variability. At that point, the fetus is probably acidotic. When the fetus is acidotic, contractions cut off the oxygen supply, and the metabolically acidotic fetal heart beats slower creating a late decel.

This flow diagram illustrates an example of a maternal cause of late decelerations.

Hypotension

Insufficient cardiac output

Decreased uterine perfusion

Deficient placental perfusion

Decreased oxygen delivery

Late deceleration(s)

ONE OR MORE LATE DECELERATIONS

There can be just one late deceleration, especially if only one contraction occurs. Frequently, a series of late decelerations are seen. Five or more late decelerations are called a *pattern of lates*. Late decelerations may occur in response to maternal hypotension. If so, accelerations and short-term variability (STV) may be seen with late decelerations. Assess the maternal blood pressure (BP). If a drug such as Ephedrine® is needed to increase BP, call the anesthesia provider.

RULES ABOUT LATE DECELERATIONS

Rules

- there can be just one late deceleration

- accelerations and short-term variability (STV) may exist, even with late decelerations (nonacidotic but hypoxic fetus)

- if there is a "shoulder" before or after the decel, it is NOT a late deceleration (it is a variable deceleration)

- late decelerations occur only in response to contractions plus oxygen deprivation

- late decels are *usually* similar in shape from one to the next

- an intrauterine pressure catheter and/or spiral electrode is NOT needed to call a deceleration a late deceleration

- a deceleration ≥ 2 minutes is a prolonged deceleration not a late deceleration.

Essentials of Fetal Monitoring

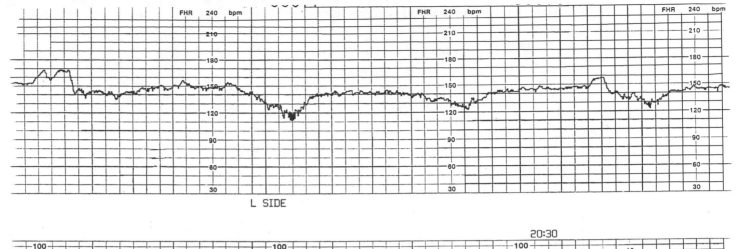

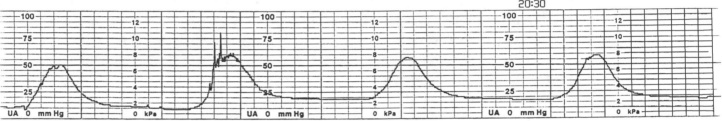

10.3   *Accelerations, short-term variability, and late decelerations.*

When late decelerations first appear, the fetus may be well-oxygenated, i.e., accelerations, movement, and STV are present.

There may be hypotension from a supine position or epidural medication. After repositioning the woman, e.g., to her side to increase cardiac output, assess blood pressure. If not contraindicated, a 500 ml bolus of lactated Ringer's (LR) solution should increase systolic blood pressure and decrease uterine activity. When 1000-1500 ml of LR has infused, cardiac output and uterine perfusion increase and contractions space out. This decrease in uterine activity and increase in cardiac output may increase fetal oxygen delivery and abolish the late decelerations. Supplemental oxygen may be needed if the late decelerations do not disappear quickly. The physician or midwife should be promptly notified. Be mindful of the complications of excessive fluid administration. Keep an accurate intake and ouptut record to avoid fluid overload.

As the hypoxic stressor continues (and late decels continue), accelerations cease. As the risk of metabolic acidosis increases, long-term variability and short-term variability decrease or become absent. The baseline may rise or fall. If there is a reactive acceleration, the fetus is hypoxic but not metabolically acidotic (see 10.3). Since the risk of metabolic acidosis is high, the FHR pattern demands prompt action to improve fetal oxygenation. As the fetus becomes more hypoxic and even acidotic you may see:

- 1st late decels
- 2nd loss of accels
- 3rd loss of long-term variability
- 4th baseline rises or falls
- 5th loss of short-term variability.

ACTIONS

Actions in Response to Late Decelerations

To improve fetal oxygenation, act to find the source of hypoxia. Also, increase *maternal blood flow* to the uterus and increase *blood oxygen content*. If the placenta is abrupting, an expeditious delivery is usually required.

The first action is to position the woman off of her back. She may lie on either her right or left side because either side improves cardiac output. Do not place her in Trendelenburg because this position decreases cardiac output. Avoid the elbows and knees (knee-chest) position if you think the uterus is rupturing because gravity may cause the fetal weight to extend an anterior uterine rupture. Once repositioned, Pitocin® and amnioinfusion should be discontinued until she is evaluated by a midwife or physician and the late decels have disappeared. Blood pressure should be assessed. If hypertension exists prior to late decelerations, position her on the side where her BP is lowest. If there are no contraindications, provide an LR fluid bolus.

Actions to Improve Maternal Blood Flow and Fetal Oxygen Delivery
• **change position**
• **discontinue oxytocin** or prostaglandins if possible
• **discontinue amnioinfusion**
• **take blood pressure**
• **provide a fluid bolus** (≥ 500 ml of lactated Ringer's solution) unless a fluid bolus is contraindicated due to an increased risk of pulmonary edema, e.g., preeclampsia or heart disease
• **administer supplemental oxygen** by a tight-fitting mask at ≥ 8 liters per minute
• **administer Ephedrine®** 5-10 mg IV push slowly over 5 minutes or as ordered for hypotension
• **terbutaline** as ordered (0.25 mg IV push slowly or subcutaneous) if there is no abruption

Essentials of Fetal Monitoring

If late decelerations started just after the amnioinfusion was initiated, discontinue the infusion. Sometimes fluid pressure on the inside uterine wall impedes oxygen delivery because vessels in the uterus are compressed.

Once the woman is on her side and Pitocin® and/or prostaglandins are discontinued, if the late decels persist, apply a tight-fitting face mask. Ask her to breathe deeply and slowly. If a simple mask is used, oxygen (O_2) should flow through the mask at 8 to 10 liters per minute. If an oxygen mask with a reservoir (partial rebreathing mask) is used, O_2 should flow at 12 liters per minute (to prevent carbon dioxide from entering the reservoir bag). A simple O_2 mask is used most often. It takes 1 to 9 minutes for oxygen to reach the fetus. Observe the FHR pattern for 10 minutes after you started oxygen. An improvement in the FHR pattern, e.g., late decels decrease in number or disappear, or accelerations reappear, indicates that the O_2 reached the fetus. Of course, a worsening of the pattern tells you otherwise, and delivery may need to be expedited. Nurses should promptly inform the midwife or physician of the FHR pattern and actions taken.

Terbutaline can mask an abruption, delay the diagnosis, and/or worsen the abruption. Therefore, prior to its use, a fully-staffed operating room crew should be present if an abruption is suspected but not ruled out.

Assess Fetal Well-being

ASSESS FETAL WELL-BEING: SCALP STIMULATION

Scalp stimulation may be done instead of scalp pH sampling. Scalp stimulation should be done **between** contractions and **between** decelerations to assess fetal acid-base status. If a $\geq$ 15 bpm x $\geq$ 15 seconds (reactive) acceleration occurs, the fetus is not yet metabolically acidotic. If a $\geq$ 10 bpm x $\geq$ 10 seconds acceleration occurs following 15 or more seconds of scalp stimulation, the fetus is not acidemic.

SCALP pH SAMPLING

Scalp pH sampling has inherent errors. pH results depend on the presence of caput, timing of the blood collection, and the physician's skill and technique. Most hospitals do not have the equipment to perform a scalp pH. A normal pH may exist even when the fetus is hypoxic. **A reactive acceleration following scalp puncture is a more accurate reflection of acid-base status than a normal pH**. Maternal hyperventilation or slow collection of the sample may result in an erroneously high pH when the fetus is actually acidotic.

SPIRAL ELECTRODE TEST

Another technique to assess fetal status is to gently pull on the spiral electrode five times, with each pull one second apart. If the fetus has a reactive acceleration within 10 seconds, metabolic acidosis is not present.

DOCUMENTATION

When you observe late decelerations, document "late decels." All late decels, regardless of their depth, represent fetal hypoxia due to uteroplacental insufficiency. Some research suggests *"The deeper the late, the lower the pH."* After documenting "late decels," record all actions, the maternal and fetal response, and your communications with the physician or midwife.

You might chart something like:

Following epidural placement, late decels noted @ 1428. Mom to L side. BP 90/58. CRNA notified. 5 mg Ephedrine® IVP per CRNA. LR IV ⇑d via IV pump. Pitocin® DCd. O₂ @ 10 LPM. 1440 no lates noted, BP 120/80. O₂ mask removed. FM (fetal movement) +, STV +. N. Nurse RNC

Another note might read:

Late decels noted @ 1700 following 5 minutes of uterine hyperstimulation. Complains of sharp, unrelenting abd pain, 5 cm blood clot noted. To R side, O₂ at 10 LPM. Dr. Caring paged to come to L & D stat. IV started in L cephalic vein with #18 1¼ inch IV cath. LR bolus initiated. Charge nurse notified of FHR pattern and suspected abruption. N. Nurse RNC

Examples of Late Decelerations

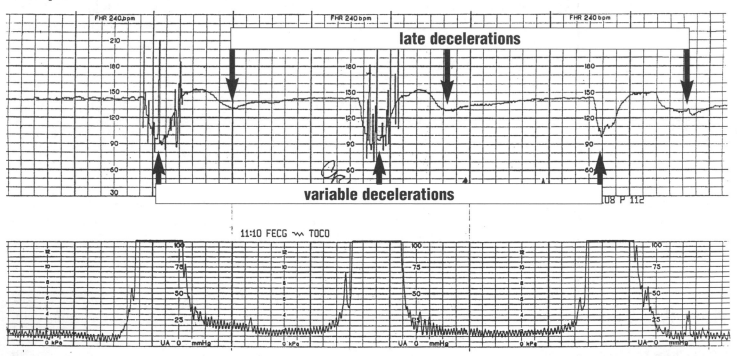

10.4 *Note that the onset to nadir duration of these late decelerations lasts 15 to 30 seconds and the contraction peak to nadir lag time is ≥ 18 seconds. When two types of decelerations occur in a repeating sequence, this is a mixed deceleration pattern or a combination or combined deceleration pattern.*

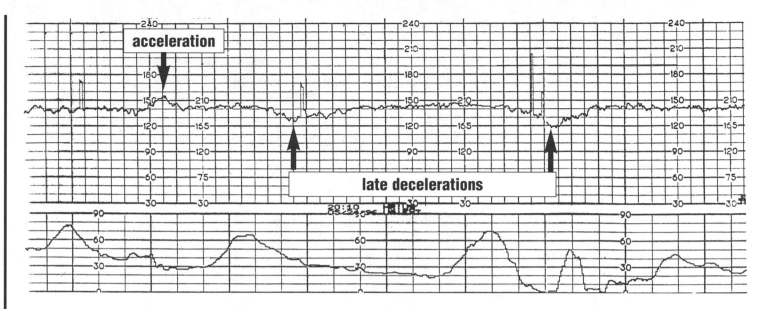

10.5 *A nearly reactive acceleration with late decelerations suggests the fetus is hypoxic but not metabolically acidotic.*

Ideally, uterine contractions appear as a waveform in the uterine activity channel. If decelerations appear but contractions are not recording on the paper, palpate for uterine activity. If there are no palpable contractions, but the decels are shaped like late decels, they are spontaneous decelerations. They reflect fetal myocardial failure, hypoxia, and/or infection and are nonreassuring. Most spontaneous decelerations are seen during antepartal fetal monitoring, especially with hypertensive women or women who are post dates with oligohydramnios. **The fetus should be delivered as soon as possible unless fetal well-being can be demonstrated, as fetuses with spontaneous decels have a high risk of intrauterine demise.**

Examples of Spontaneous Deceleration

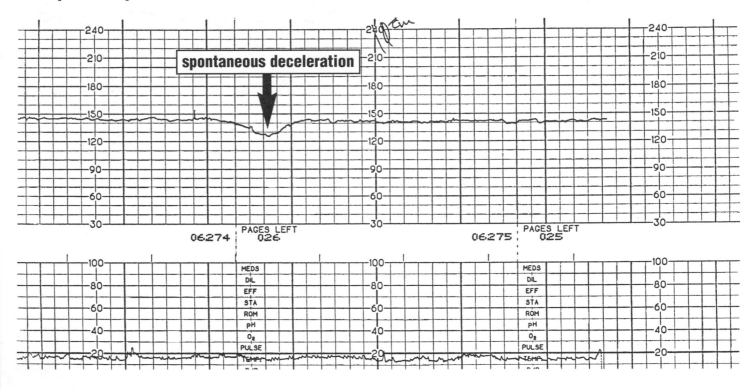

10.6 *Spontaneous decelerations are not late decelerations. They occur when there are no contractions, often in fetuses of hypertensive women. They reflect fetal myocardial failure and may be a response to fetal hypoxia or infection. In this case, there was hypertension, oligohydramnios, and intrauterine growth restriction. Apgar scores were 1, 3, and 5 at 1, 5, and 10 minutes.*

CORD/ PLACENTAL GASES

To confirm the fetal and placental status just prior to birth, blood gases may be obtained. Umbilical cord or placental blood can be sampled. Arterial blood gases reflect fetal status and venous blood gases reflect placental status prior to birth. A syringe flushed with 1000 U/ml heparin may be used. Using 10,000U/ml heparin produces erroneous results. Usually only 1 ml of blood is needed but it is best to ask laboratory personnel what they need. The blood gases are stable in the syringe at room temperature up to one hour after their collection. However, laboratory standards require the blood be analyzed within 60 minutes after their collection. Laboratory personnel like the syringe to be placed in a slush of ice, even though the ice has no effect on test results. Ask an experienced clinician to show you how to obtain blood gas samples.

PLACENTAL PATHOLOGY

Since an abnormal placenta may be the primary cause of uteroplacental insufficiency, it may be helpful to send the placenta to pathology. On the pathology request, include pertinent risk or history information and indications for the pathology study. The physician may request **center cuts** of the placenta or **cross cut sections** of the umbilical cord. These requests ensure quality slides for accurate placental diagnosis. If meconium is present, do *not* place the placenta in formalin because it dissolves meconium pigment and may change the pathology results. If the newborn has meconium staining, document on the newborn record a description of the meconium staining and color, e.g., yellow fingernails, yellow vernix, or green cord. The color, amount, and odor of the amniotic fluid should also be recorded in the woman's record.

Reflex Late Decelerations

Dr. Julian Parer has suggested there are two kinds of late deceleration patterns: reflex late decelerations and hypoxic myocardial failure late decelerations. The presence or absence of short-term variability determines which exists.

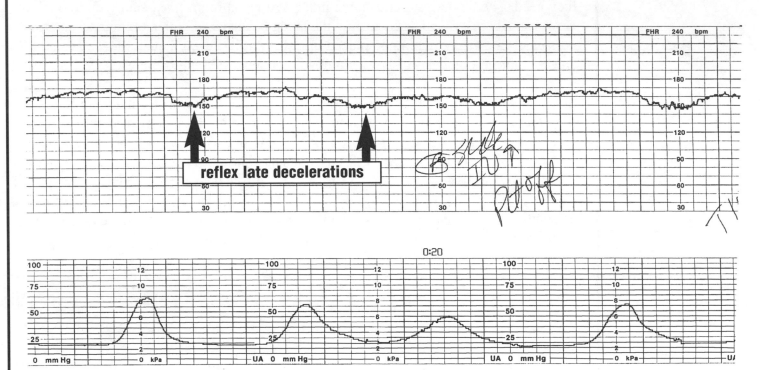

10.7   *Short-term variability in the baseline suggests the fetus is hypoxic but not metabolically acidotic. These are reflex late decelerations. Note the contraction peak to deceleration nadir lag time is ≥ 18 seconds. The baseline is tachycardic. Appropriate actions were to position the woman on her right side, increase the intravenous fluid flow rate, discontinue Pitocin®, and call the midwife and/or physician. Document "late decels, STV+, LTV absent-av."*

A reflex late decel is a chemoreceptor-vagal response to hypoxia. There is usually a stable baseline with short-term variability. The offset of reflex late decelerations may be gradual or abrupt. Accels may precede or follow this type of late deceleration pattern. The fetus is hypoxic but not metabolically acidotic.

Hypoxic Myocardial Failure Late Decelerations

When late decels occur and short-term variability is absent, the fetus has hypoxic myocardial failure late decelerations and is probably metabolically acidotic and should be promptly delivered.

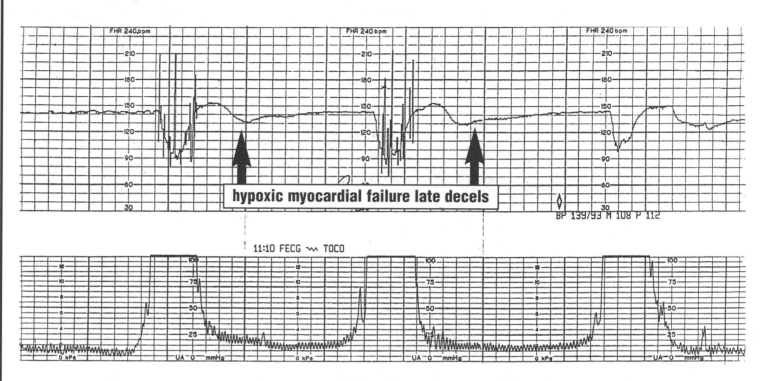

10.8 *Hypoxic myocardial failure late decelerations. This child suffered permanent, irreversible brain damage and has cerebral palsy. Document "late decels, 0 LTV, 0 STV" and expedite delivery.*

Summary

Late decelerations are periodic decelerations associated with hypoxia. They have a slanted onset, reaching their nadir in as little as 15 seconds but often in 30 or more seconds. They may have a boxy, U, V, or saucer shape. They last less than 2 minutes. If short-term variability is present or accelerations are present the fetus is hypoxic but not metabolically acidotic. These are classified as reflex late decelerations but are documented as "late decelerations, STV present." If short-term variability is absent, the pattern of late decelerations reflects metabolic acidosis and has been called hypoxic myocardial failure late decelerations. They are documented as "late decelerations, STV absent." Whenever late decelerations occur, actions to improve oxygen delivery to the fetus should be initiated. These may include a position change, discontinuing uterine stimulants and amnioinfusion, blood pressure assessment, giving Ephedrine® as ordered, administering an intravenous bolus of lactated Ringer's solution, oxygen by a tight-fitting face mask, and terbutaline as ordered provided there is no abruption. Terbutaline can mask an abruption or extend the abruption. Oxygen should reach the fetus within 9 minutes. Document late decelerations and other FHR pattern characteristics, all actions, communications, and the fetal and maternal response.

SECTION 10:   LATE DECELERATIONS

QUESTIONS

Directions: Circle T if the statement is true, F if it is false.

QUESTIONS

T   F   1.   Late decelerations all have a gradual onset and offset.

T   F   2.   All late decelerations begin at or after the peak of the contraction.

T   F   3.   Late decelerations are often similar in shape.

T   F   4.   If short-term variability is present, they are not late decelerations.

T   F   5.   If accelerations are present, they are not late decelerations.

T   F   6.   It takes 15 minutes for supplemental oxygen to reach the fetus.

T   F   7.   Hypotension may precede late decelerations.

T   F   8.   Late decelerations may last more than 2 minutes.

T   F   9.   Late decelerations are indicative of fetal hypoxia.

Essentials of Fetal Monitoring

SECTION 11
Variable Decelerations (Variable decels)

Pressure on	Type of Deceleration
• fetal head	• early
• uterine vessels	• late
• **umbilical cord**	• **variable**

Variable decelerations vary in shape, depth, and duration and can occur during or between contractions.

DEFINITION AND RECOGNITION CRITERIA OF A VARIABLE DECELERATION

A variable deceleration is a U, V, or W shaped drop in the fetal heart rate with a duration of 15 or more seconds and a descent of 15 or more bpm. The deceleration duration is the time between the onset of the descent and the recovery *at the baseline level*. A prompt recovery is a nadir to baseline time of 8 to 27 seconds. Since it is hard to see 27 seconds, a slow recovery is one that takes 30 or more seconds from nadir to baseline.

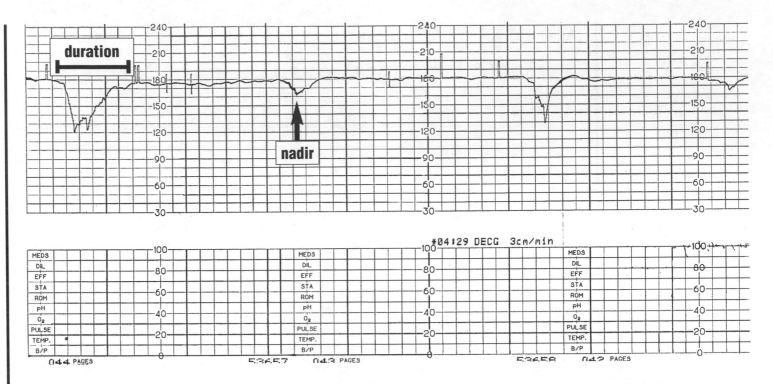

11.1 *The nadir is the lowest point of a deceleration. This is an example of variable decelerations, tachycardia, absent to minimal long-term variability, absent short-term variability, and absent accelerations. This is a nonreassuring pattern.*

Anything smaller than 15 bpm x 15 seconds is called a "dip." Dips are common in preterm fetuses, but all fetuses have "dips" in their fetal heart rate. Dips have no clinical significance.

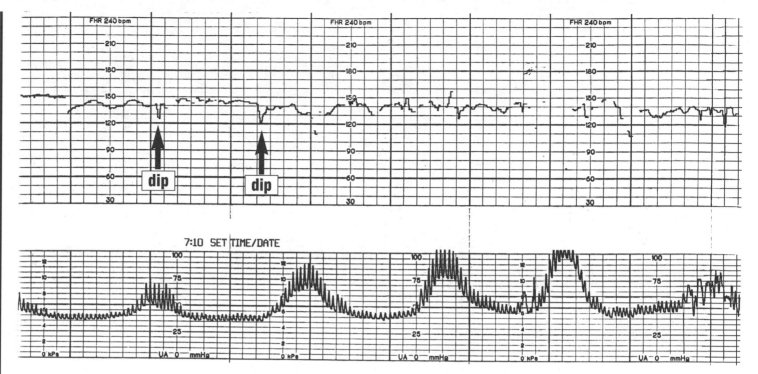

11.2   There are multiple dips present, but not decelerations. This fetus was 26 weeks of gestation and was delivered preterm. "Set time/date" reflects a need for a new clock battery.

The clinical significance of a variable deceleration depends on the stability of the baseline, the presence or absence of baseline long-term variability (LTV) and short-term variability (STV), the presence of accelerations, and the timing of the deceleration, i.e., with or between uterine contractions.

Variable decelerations are usually a response to umbilical cord compression. Variable decels usually abruptly fall and recover. **The lack of accelerations and/or STV is more significant and concerning than a prompt or slow recovery.**

During vein and artery compression in the umbilical cord, there is an increase in fetal blood pressure, a decrease in fetal PaO_2, an increase in $PaCO_2$, and a decrease in pH, which activates specialized nerves called baroreceptors and chemoreceptors. This triggers a vagal response. Usually there is a prompt return to baseline. However, when recovery is slow, lasting 30 or more seconds, there is even greater concern that the fetus is more hypoxic and needs supplemental oxygen. Act to relieve umbilical cord compression, improve uterine perfusion, and improve maternal blood oxygen content.

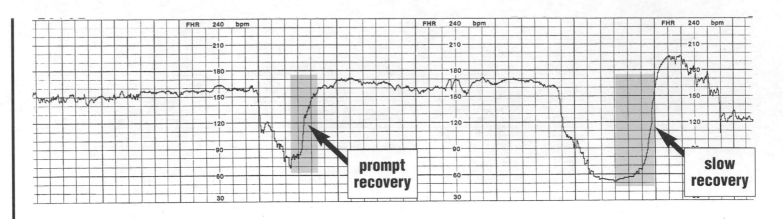

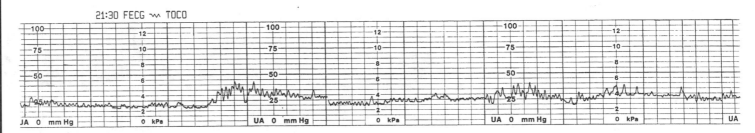

11.3 *Recovery (from the nadir to the baseline) is prompt when the recovery is < 30 seconds and is slow if it is ≥ 30 seconds. This illustration shows each type of recovery. Actions to decrease cord compression and increase maternal cardiac output, uterine perfusion, and blood oxygen content should be instituted. Communicate promptly with the midwife or physician.*

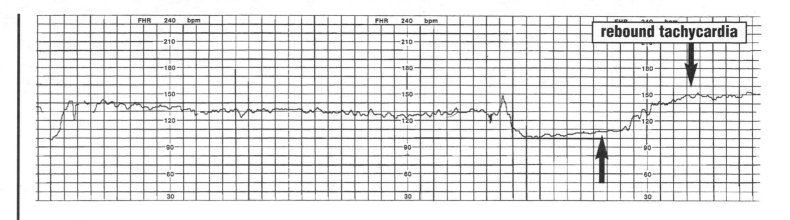

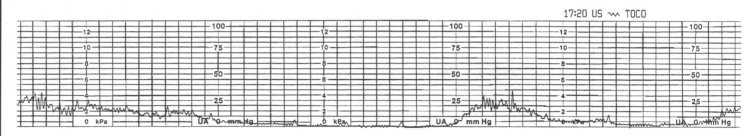

11.4   *Slow recovery of a variable deceleration reflects a slow cardiac recovery from hypoxia and an increased risk of fetal metabolic acidosis. Notice the rebound tachycardia. Catecholamines have increased the fetal blood pressure and heart rate.*

SHAPES OF VARIABLE DECELERATIONS

A variable deceleration is a transient decrease in the FHR with a U, V, or W shape. The W shape has been associated with a cord that is 50 cm or longer. (See 11.5, 11.6, and 11.7).

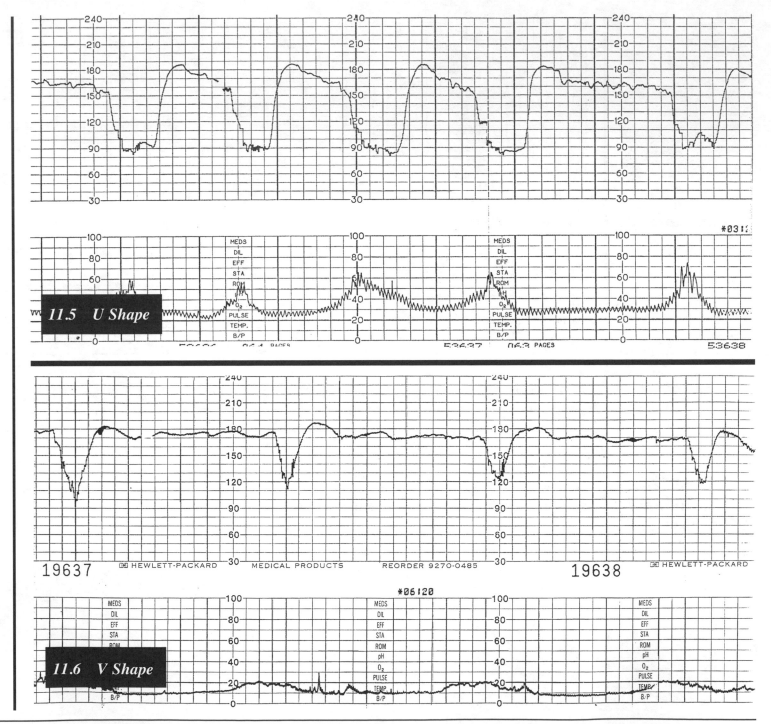

11.5   U Shape

11.6   V Shape

Essentials of Fetal Monitoring

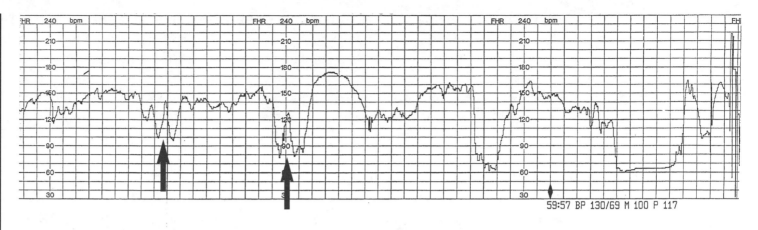

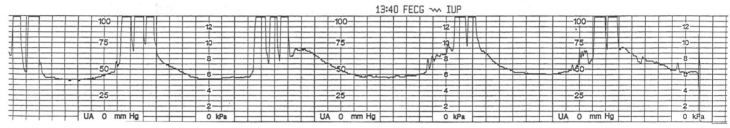

11.7   W Shape

The depth and duration of a variable deceleration are less predictive of Apgar scores or fetal scalp pH than the presence or absence of baseline short-term variability. The incidence of low Apgars and a compromised neonate increases when there is, in addition to variable decels,

- tachycardia

- bradycardia

- decreased or absent long-term and short-term variability

- presence of atypical variable deceleration features and/or the

- absence of accelerations.

The fetus who has any deceleration to a rate less than 80 bpm has an increased risk of hypoxia. As the FHR falls, so does the fetal blood pressure, and the fetus' ability to perfuse its brain decreases. In illustration 11.3 the decelerations fell to 52 to 70 beats per minute and were less than 80 bpm for up to almost 50 seconds during the second deceleration. Hypoxia is reflected by the slow recovery and an overshoot. The fetus in this illustration is attempting to compensate. Epinephrine and norepinephrine, which are released by the adrenal glands, produce the overshoot. Overshoots are part of a nonreassuring pattern.

TYPICAL VARIABLE DECELERATIONS HAVE "SHOULDERS"

Typical variable decelerations are also known as classic or pure variable decelerations. They have "shoulders" on either side of the variable deceleration. "Shoulders" are also called "an acceleratory phase of the deceleration pattern." They are part of the deceleration and are **not** accelerations.

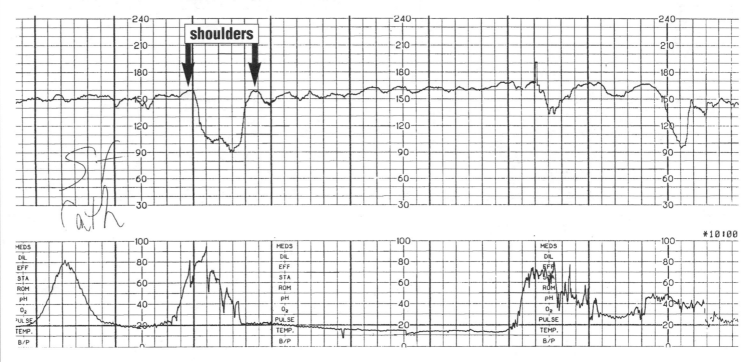

11.8   Classic variable decelerations with "shoulders."

A shoulder, which is an increase in the FHR preceding and/or following a variable deceleration, is a fetal response to umbilical **vein** compression. It is a sign that the fetus is trying to compensate for the slight drop in PaO_2 and BP during mild cord compression.

OVERSHOOTS

A nonreassuring sign is an increase in the size or duration of the secondary "shoulder" following a variable deceleration. Shoulders are usually no higher than 20 bpm above the baseline and are less than or equal to 20 seconds in duration. *An overshoot may be more than 20 bpm above the baseline or last longer than 20 seconds.*

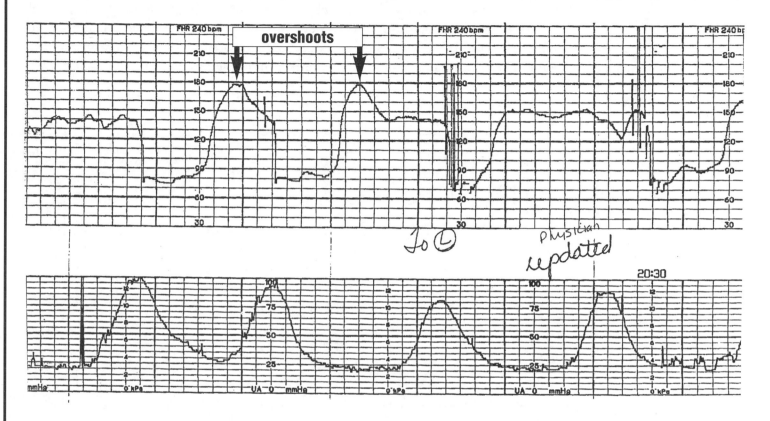

11.9   Two overshoots following variable decelerations. Note uterine hyperstimulation. Actions to decrease uterine activity and relieve cord compression, such as a position change to the left side, are needed.

Overshoots suggest fetal hypoxia. Actions to improve fetal oxygenation are needed. Overshoots are **not** accelerations. Recurring variable decelerations with overshoots are **not** a reassuring sign. They are associated with a low fetal pH. Look at the baseline. If short-term variability is present, it rules out metabolic acidosis but not hypoxia. Since overshoots are nonreassuring, the midwife and/or physician should be promptly informed.

Atypical Variable Decelerations

Atypical variable decelerations are identified by their shape. Some atypical variable decelerations are missing one or both shoulders. Others look smooth. The significance of a pattern depends on the presence of baseline short-term variability, accelerations, and a baseline in a normal range. Atypical variable decelerations during the 30 minutes preceding birth often reflect significant fetal hypoxia with a PO_2 less than 15 mm Hg. Atypical variable deceleration features suggest an increased risk of fetal hypoxia, especially in combination with a smooth deceleration, tachycardia, bradycardia, and/or a deceleration duration of 45 or more seconds.

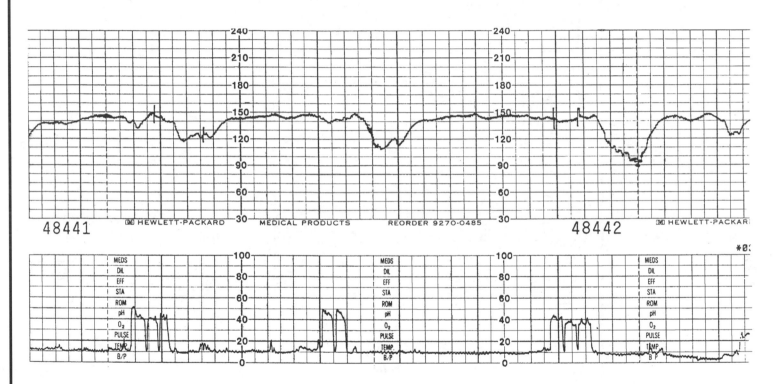

11.10 Atypical feature: loss of initial and secondary shoulders. Note the absence of long-term and short-term variability, and the lack of accelerations.

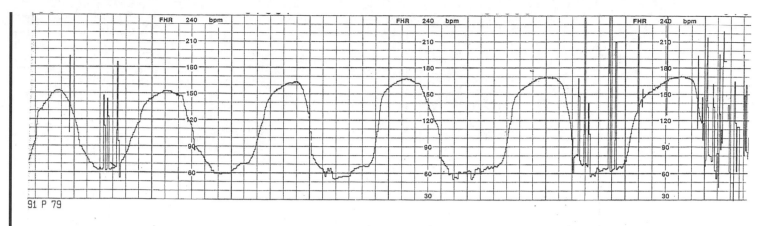

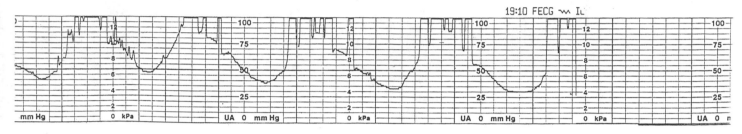

11.11   Atypical feature: smooth decelerations. Note uterine hyperstimulation, hypertonus, and pushing during contractions.

Smooth atypical variable decelerations precede low Apgar scores. The smooth decelerations in this example are additionally significant because of the slow recovery and overshoots. There is less than one minute between contractions. This is an inadequate amount of time to reoxygenate the fetus. Fetal decompensation and newborn resusitation are highly probable following this nonreassuring pattern.

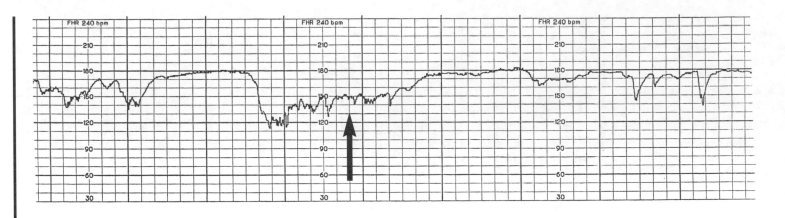

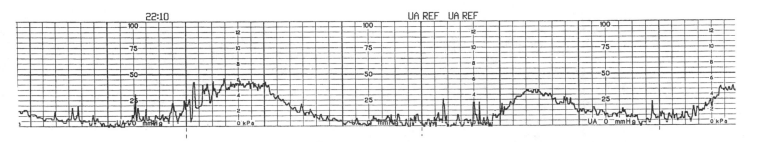

11.12 *Atypical feature: continuation of the baseline at a lower level. Note at about 2211 a variable deceleration to 115 bpm, followed by a baseline at 140-150 bpm that increases to the 170s. The baseline increases to 180 bpm. Fetal acidemia should be ruled out when there is tachycardia and variable decelerations, especially when short-term variability is absent or nearly absent. If well-being cannot be confirmed following actions to improve fetal oxygenation, the delivery should be expedited and newborn resusitation should be anticipated.*

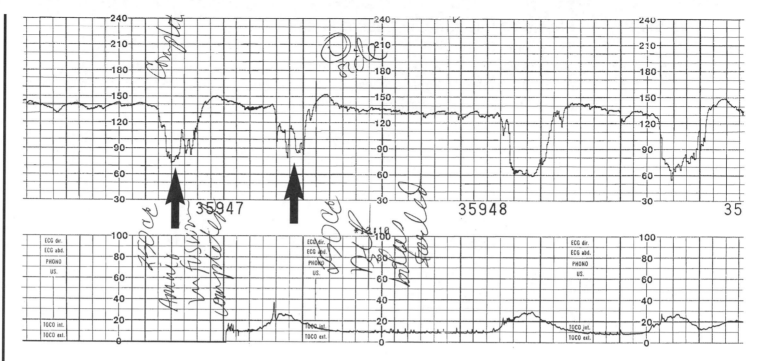

11.13 Atypical feature: biphasic variable deceleration or W shape.

A W shaped variable deceleration is also called a biphasic variable and is considered atypical. However, the W shape is not as significant in predicting fetal status as the baseline rate, short-term variability, and accelerations. A W shaped decel with accelerations and a normal baseline and variability is reassuring. A W shaped decel with tachycardia, no accelerations, and decreased to absent variability is nonreassuring.

CLASSIFICATION OF VARIABLE DECELERATIONS

Classification of Variable Decelerations

How you document variable decelerations will depend on your hospital's chart forms. Some chart forms provide criteria for mild, moderate, and severe variable decels.

It is essential to record the duration and depth of variable decelerations if there is no chart form legend.

	Duration	Depth
Mild variable deceleration:	< 30 seconds	any depth but not < 70 to 80 bpm
Moderate variable deceleration:	30-60 seconds	usually not < 70 bpm
Severe variable deceleration:	> 60 seconds	may be < 70 bpm

Physiology of Variable Decelerations

The depth of variable decelerations indirectly reflects the degree of fetal hypotension and the fetal response to cord compression. The decelerations are caused by slowing of sinoatrial nodal impulses. As the fetal heart rate drops, the fetal blood pressure also drops. This might decrease fetal brain perfusion. Fetal oxygen can become depleted. The longer a variable deceleration lasts, the higher the risk becomes of fetal metabolic acidosis.

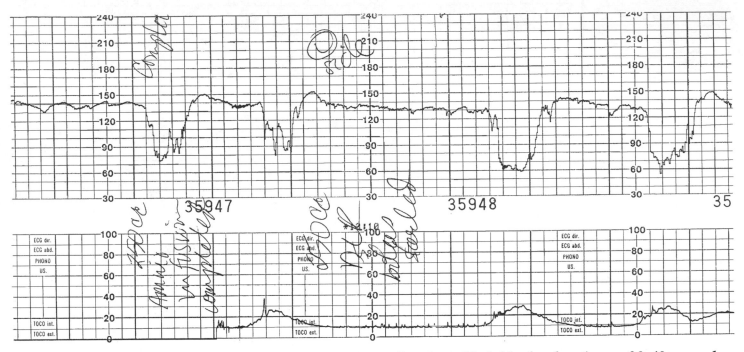

11.13   Baseline 130-142, LTV absent to average. No accelerations. Variable decelerations x 30-40 seconds ⇓ 60-85 bpm. Amnioinfusion was completed and an IV bolus of D₅LR was started. The woman was placed on her left side. Which intervention was inappropriate?

Actions in Response to Variable Decelerations

The response to variable decelerations depends on where the fetus lies on the continuum between well-oxygenated and asphyxiated. An IV bolus may help decrease uterine activity but plain LR, not D₅LR, should be used because D₅LR can precipitate newborn hypoglycemia.

Variable decelerations are usually due to umbilical cord compression. However, head compression during the second stage, may make variable decelerations deeper.

Possible Nursing Actions for Cord Compression

- change maternal position and observe the fetal response

- perform a vaginal exam to rule out imminent delivery or cord prolapse

- begin amnioinfusion if ordered

- hyperoxygenate with a simple face mask at 8-10 L/minute or a partial rebreathing mask at 12 L/minute

- observe for an improvement within 1 to 9 minutes

- communicate and document assessments and interventions to the midwife and/or physician

- infuse ≥ 500 ml lactated Ringer's solution to decrease uterine activity.

DOCUMENTATION

Documentation

Variable decelerations vary in configuration, duration, and depth. Document the range of variable decel durations in seconds and depths in bpm. If more than one variable deceleration is present, the range of durations and depths is recorded, e.g., "variable decels 35-45 seconds, ⇓ 80-110 bpm." If the recovery is slow (≥ 30 seconds) it would be important to document it, e.g., "return to baseline x 45 seconds." This slow return to baseline is indicative of worsening hypoxia, and nursing interventions should include hyperoxygenation with a tight-fitting face mask. Usually, "atypical" is not used in documentation to describe variable decelerations. Document *compensatory signs* such as "variable decelerations *with primary shoulder*" or signs of fetal well-being such as "STV present, spont. accels ⇑ 170 x 30 sec."

SUMMARY

Summary

Variable decelerations are transient decreases in the FHR. They have U, V or W shapes. Variable decelerations last at least 15 seconds and decrease 15 or more beats per minute. The fetal heart rate abruptly falls (usually at the nadir in less than 30 seconds), the depth varies, and the return to baseline usually is abrupt (8-27 seconds). However, if the return to baseline is slow (≥ 30 seconds), it suggests a hypoxic fetus with myocardial depression. Tachycardia and/or decreased or absent variability with variable decelerations are related to fetal acidemia.

The primary and secondary acceleratory phases of the variable deceleration pattern (shoulders) are a compensatory response to umbilical vein compression. When a variable deceleration is preceded and followed by a shoulder it is considered a classic, pure, or "typical" variable deceleration. When one or both "shoulders" are missing, the deceleration is smooth, the baseline after the deceleration is lower, there is an overshoot, or the variable decel has a W shape, the deceleration is called atypical. If the deceleration falls below 80 bpm, fetal brain perfusion is compromised. Act to improve umbilical cord blood flow and oxygen delivery to the fetus.

SECTION 11: VARIABLE DECELERATIONS

QUESTIONS

QUESTIONS

Directions: Circle T if the statement is true, F if it is false.

T   F   1.   Variable decelerations are uniform in shape and size.

T   F   2.   Variable decelerations are only a periodic pattern, they are never nonperiodic.

T   F   3.   Expect very low Apgar scores when there are variable decelerations, absent long-term variability and absent short-term variability.

T   F   4.   An atypical feature of a variable deceleration is a shoulder.

T   F   5.   An overshoot is an increase in the fetal heart rate following a variable deceleration. The increase is 15 bpm above the baseline which lasts 15 seconds.

T   F   6.   A low fetal pH is associated with repetitive variable decelerations with overshoots.

T   F   7.   A biphasic variable deceleration is related to an umbilical cord less than 50 cm in length.

T   F   8.   Utilizing descriptors of mild, moderate, and severe adequately documents variable decelerations.

T   F   9.   A variable deceleration nadir less than 80 bpm has no clinical significance.

T   F   10.   Variable decelerations lasting 60 or more seconds and falling to less than 70 bpm are associated with fetal acidemia.

SECTION 12
Prolonged Decelerations

PROLONGED DECELERATION DEFINITION

A prolonged deceleration is a deceleration that lasts 2 to 10 minutes. It usually has an abrupt onset and a gradual recovery. If the fetal heart rate stays down for 10 or more minutes, bradycardia begins and a prolonged deceleration ends. Document the deceleration duration and nadir depth rather than "prolonged decel."

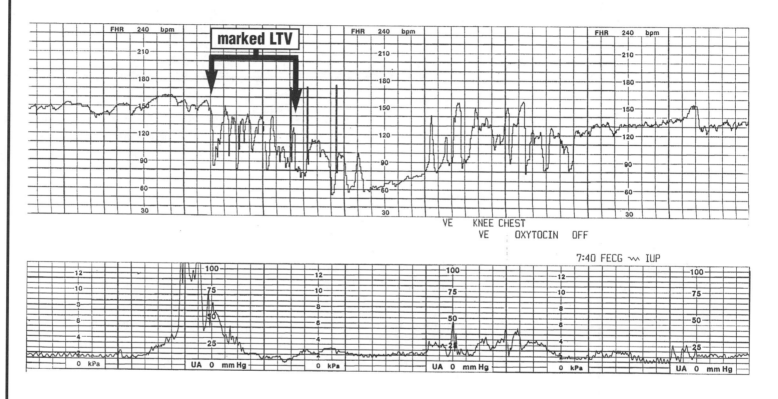

12.1 *Document this as "decel x 5 minutes ⇓ 60 bpm." Note short-term variability and a 15 second spontaneous acceleration are present after the prolonged deceleration. The presence of marked long-term variability during the first minute suggests this prolonged deceleration was due to umbilical cord compression. Note the appropriate actions of a position change (knee-chest), a vaginal examination (VE) to rule out a cord prolapse, and discontinuation of oxytocin.*

Determine the etiology of the prolonged decel. Usually it's maternal hypotension or umbilical cord compression.

CAUSES OF PROLONGED DECELERATIONS

Causes of Prolonged Decelerations	
Maternal Causes	Fetal Causes
• hypotension • excessive uterine activity • seizure	• umbilical cord compression • hypoxia, e.g., due to maternal hypotension or uterine hyperstimulation • direct anesthetic response

As long as tissue oxygen (O_2) is present, fetal hypoxemia will not progress to tissue hypoxia, acidemia or acidosis. Fetal O_2 is depleted when the FHR is less than 80 bpm. An FHR less than 80 bpm is a reflection of fetal hypotension and decreased fetal brain perfusion. When fetal O_2 becomes depleted, metabolic acidosis can occur. The evidence of metabolic acidosis is the absence of short-term variability, long-term variability, and accelerations. **Following a prolonged deceleration and subsequent metabolic acidosis, the FHR will become bradycardic and may be an agonal pattern or terminal bradycardia from which the fetus will not recover.**

REBOUND TACHYCARDIA

Fetal tachycardia following a deceleration is reflective of a catecholamine and hypertensive response to hypoxia, and is called rebound tachycardia. The fetus has peripheral vasoconstriction and is increasing blood flow to the brain, heart, and adrenal glands (vital organs). This is *not* a reassuring sign. It is a compensatory sign. While one prolonged deceleration may be a fetal compensatory response to a temporary asphyxial insult, two or more prolonged decelerations are nonreassuring and raise one's suspicion of such causes as occult cord prolapse, hypotension, and/or a need to expedite delivery by cesarean section.

Actions in Response to a Prolonged Deceleration

- turn the woman to her side to maximize maternal cardiac output and umbilical cord blood flow

- discontinue uterine stimulants

- discontinue amnioinfusion if the pattern worsened after initiating amnioinfusion

- decrease uterine activity by infusing ≥ 500 ml of lactated Ringer's (LR) solution

- administer Ephedrine® 5 to 10 mg slow IV push if it is ordered for maternal hypotension

- hyperoxygenate maternal plasma, provide oxygen by a tight-fitting face mask at 8-10 or 12 liters per minute depending on mask type

- perform a vaginal examination to rule out imminent delivery and/or cord prolapse

- administer a tocolytic if it is ordered by the physician or midwife and the placenta is not abrupting

- communicate with the charge nurse, midwife and/or physician.

To gently flush the vagina of intravaginal prostaglandin gel, you may attach a catheter to a 20 cc syringe filled with normal saline and irrigate the vagina or attach IV tubing to a small bag of normal saline, insert the tubing into the vagina, and infuse the fluid. A rapid response is needed when a prolonged deceleration appears, but a cesarean section may not be needed unless an abruption or a uterine rupture is suspected. If you suspect uterine rupture, turn her to her side, do **not** place the woman in a knee-chest position. Notify the midwife or physician of the deceleration, your assessments, and actions.

EVALUATE FETAL STATUS AND DOCUMENT

Evaluate Fetal Status and Document

After a prolonged deceleration, the fetus needs to be resuscitated within the uterus if possible. This is called **intrauterine resuscitation**.

- Did a position change help? Document the response of the fetus.

- Evaluate the strip for evidence of fetal well-being. Is the amniotic fluid clear and nonfoul?

- What was the dilatation, effacement, and station?

- Has the FHR recovered to its previous baseline or is it higher than before?

- Document communication with the other nurses, physician or midwife, and notification of the neonatal resuscitation team.

- Document signs of fetal well-being beyond a stable FHR such as:
  - accelerations
  - short-term variability
  - fetal movement.

- A prolonged deceleration may reoccur.
  - Discontinue uterine stimulants until the midwife and/or physician have evaluated the woman and the fetus.
  - Is a tocolytic necessary?

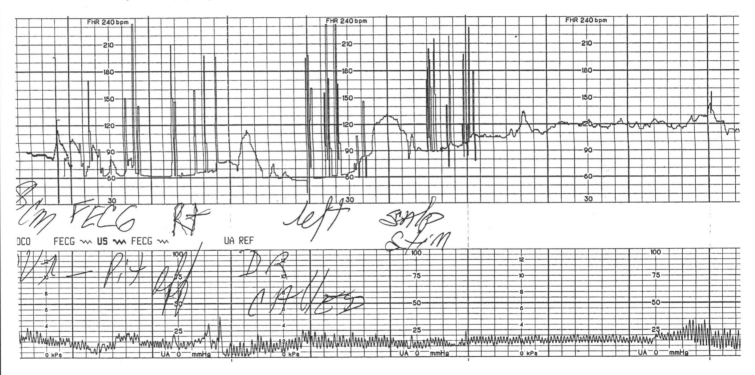

12.2 *Scalp stimulation is NOT useful during a fetal deceleration or bradycardia because the vagal response overrides any sympathetic nerve stimulus.*

SCALP STIMULATION IS AN ASSESSMENT METHOD NOT AN INTERVENTION

Scalp stimulation during a deceleration is inappropriate. It may create a vagal response. It delays appropriate actions. The fetus needs oxygen not touch. Scalp stimulation should be done between contractions and between decelerations when there is a clear baseline, to elicit an acceleration and rule out metabolic acidosis.

Summary

A prolonged deceleration lasts 2 to 10 minutes. Its duration and depth are documented instead of using the words "prolonged deceleration." The most common cause of prolonged decelerations is umbilical cord compression. Some prolonged decelerations occur as a result of maternal hypotension and transient fetal hypoxia. Actions to improve fetal oxygen delivery are done first, e.g., a position change. Avoid the knee-chest position if a uterine rupture is suspected. You may choose to administer an intravenous bolus of a non-glucose solution, discontinue the Pitocin® drip and/or amnioinfusion, and administer supplemental oxygen. Actions are also directed at determining the cause of the prolonged deceleration. These include assessing blood pressure and a vaginal examination to rule out an umbilical cord prolapse. If hyperstimulation is evident, oxytocics are discontinued or intravaginal prostaglandins are flushed from the vagina. Communicate assessments and actions to the charge nurse, the midwife and/or physician. Document the signs of fetal well-being following the prolonged deceleration. Signs of fetal well-being include accelerations, short-term variability, and fetal movement. Scalp stimulation during the deceleration is **not** appropriate. This assessment technique is used, in place or scalp pH sampling, to rule out metabolic acidosis after the deceleration. It is done **between** decelerations and **between** contractions.

SECTION 12: PROLONGED DECELERATIONS

QUESTIONS

Directions: Circle T if the statement is true, F if it is false.

QUESTIONS

T   F   1.   A prolonged deceleration lasts 2 to 15 minutes.

T   F   2.   Fetal tachycardia following fetal bradycardia is a reassuring sign.

T   F   3.   A prolonged deceleration may be due to fetal head compression.

T   F   4.   Maternal hypotension may precede a prolonged deceleration.

T   F   5.   Actions during a prolonged deceleration include fetal scalp stimulation.

T   F   6.   Following a prolonged deceleration, the return to a baseline within the normal range in and of itself is reassuring.

T   F   7.   Supplemental oxygen is not useful when a prolonged deceleration occurs.

T   F   8.   The presence of baseline long-term variability in and of itself following a prolonged deceleration confirms fetal well-being.

T   F   9.   Two or more prolonged decelerations represent a nonreassuring fetal heart rate pattern.

SECTION 13
Strip Evaluation and Categorization

In this section, you will evaluate your knowlege and visual assessment skill. Fill in the blanks after each question then look at the correct responses on pages 185 and 186. Remember, visual assessment rarely has 100% agreement, so the numbers we state as correct may be slightly different from yours.

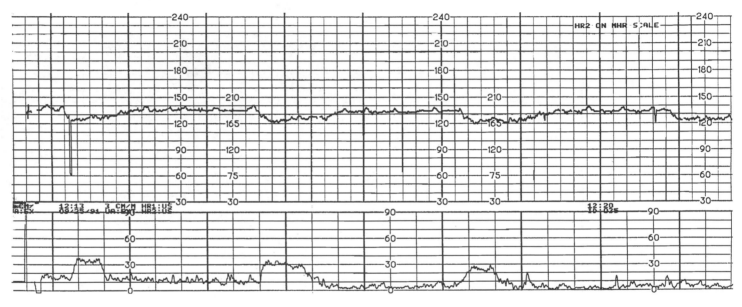

13.1   Strip 1.

1. What is the FHR at the nadirs in bpm? _____-_____ bpm

2. Is the contraction peak-to-deceleration nadir lag time greater or less than 18 seconds? _____

3. What is the recovery time from nadir to baseline? _____-_____ seconds

4. What kind of decelerations are these?

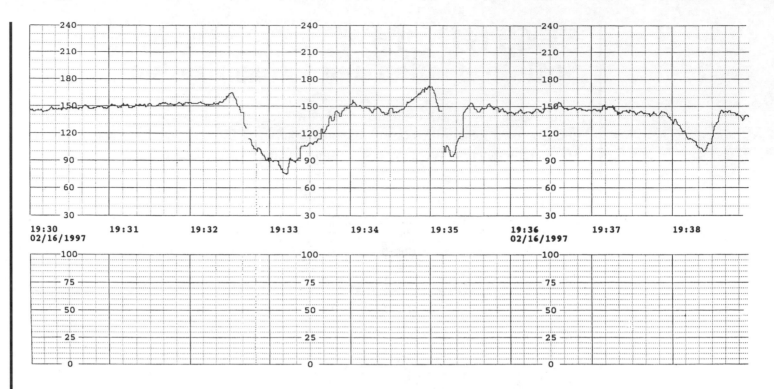

13.2 Strip 2.

5. What is the duration of the decelerations in seconds? _____-_____ seconds

6. What is the depth of the nadirs in bpm? _____-_____ bpm

7. What is the recovery time from nadir to baseline? _____-_____ seconds

8. What kind of decelerations are these?

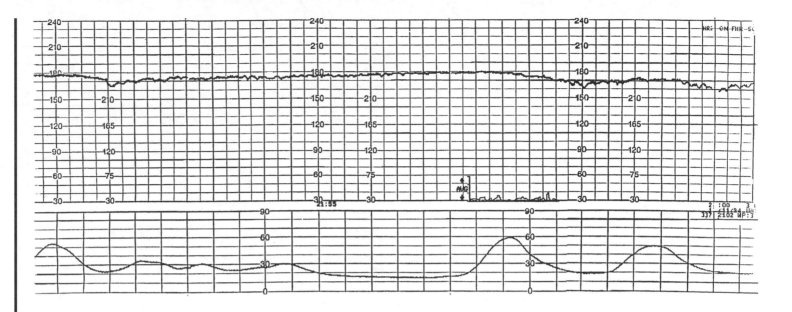

13.3   Strip 3.

9.   How long is the onset from baseline to nadir? _____ seconds

10.   What is the lag time between the contraction peak and the nadirs in seconds? _____-_____ seconds

11.   What is the recovery time from nadir to baseline? _____ seconds

12.   What kind of decelerations are these?

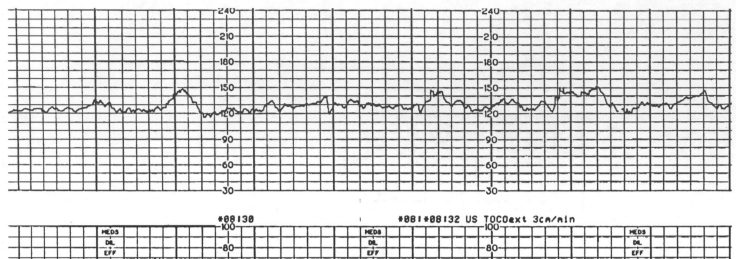

13.4 Strip 4.

13. What is the baseline range? _____ - _____ bpm

14. Is short-term variability present or absent? _____

15. Classify long-term variability. _____

16. What is the FHR at the height of the accelerations? _____ - _____ bpm

17. What is the duration of the accelerations? _____ - _____ seconds

18. Are any of these reactive accelerations? ❏ Yes or ❏ No

19. Is this fetus metabolically acidotic? ❏ Yes or ❏ No

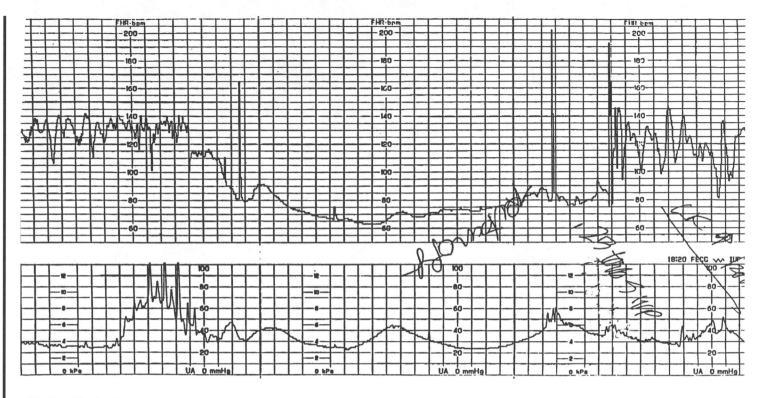

13.5 Strip 5.

20. Is this a periodic or episodic (nonperiodic) deceleration? _____

21. What is the duration of the deceleration? _____ minutes

22. What is the FHR at the nadir of the deceleration? _____ bpm

23. What are the two most likely causes of this deceleration?

      1. _____   2. _____

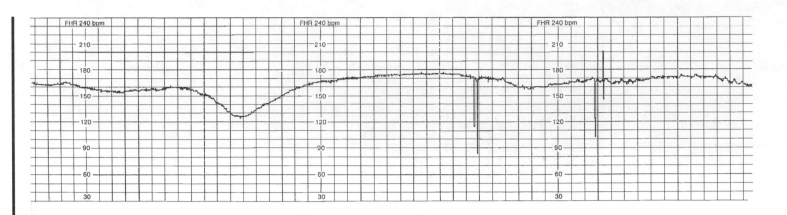

5:40 FECG ᴍ IUP

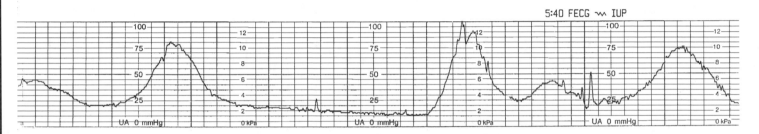

13.6   Strip 6.

24.   What kind of decelerations are these? _____

25.   What is the contraction frequency? every _____ minute(s)

26.   What is the contraction duration? _____-_____ seconds

27.   What is the contraction strength/peak intrauterine pressure? _____-_____ mm Hg

28.   What is the resting tone? _____-_____ mm Hg

29.   What is this uterine activity called? _____

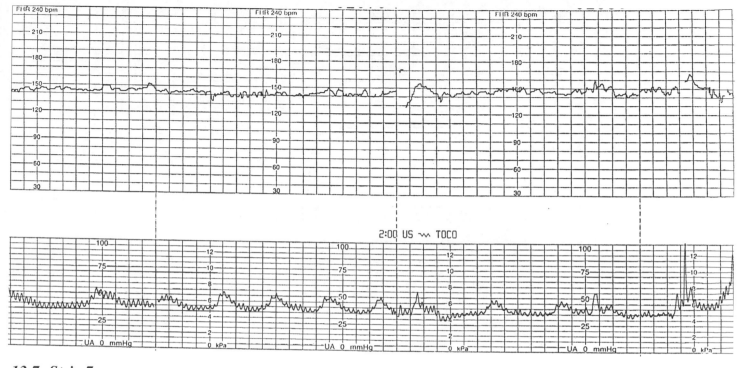

13.7 Strip 7.

30. What would you record as the baseline? _____ - _____ bpm

31. Classify STV. STV is _____

32. Classify LTV. LTV is _____

33. Are there any accelerations?_____

34. Are there any decelerations?_____

35. Is this normal UA?_____

36. If no, what is this called? _____

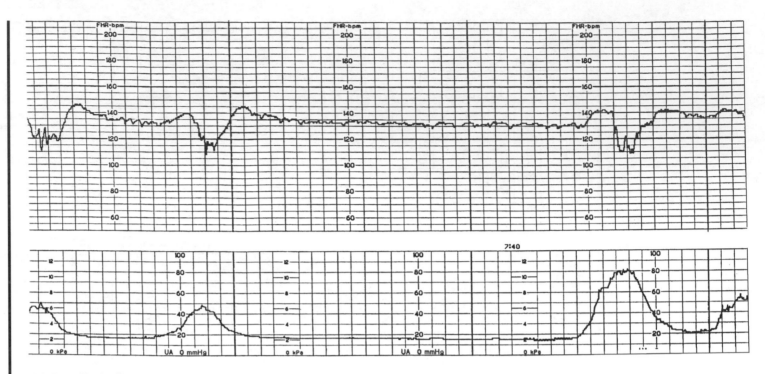

13.8   Strip 8.

37.   Fill in each box for Strip 8

BL	STV	LTV	Accels	Decels
			ht _____ bpm duration _____ sec	type _____ duration _____ sec depth _____ bpm

38.   What is the most likely cause of this pattern?

    a.   head compression

    b.   cord compression

    c.   inadequate uteroplacental perfusion

39. What actions would you take in response to this pattern (13.8)? (Circle the letter of all that apply)

a. do nothing, it's a normal fetal response

b. turn the woman

c. discontinue Pitocin®

d. increase IV fluids

e. observe the pattern

f. apply oxygen by mask

g. notify the midwife or doctor

h. perform a vaginal examination

i. take maternal blood pressure

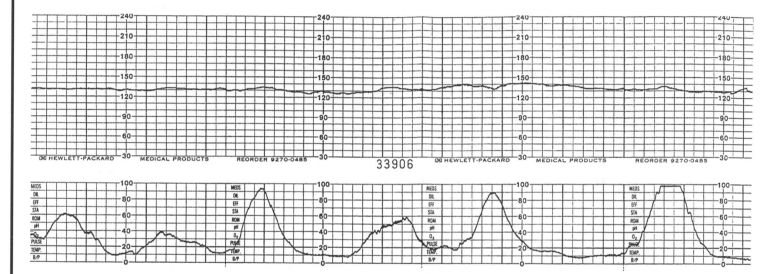

33906

13.9 Strip 9.

Fill in each box for strip 9. Demerol 25 mg IV push was administered 10 minutes ago. Prior to the pattern the fetal heart rate pattern was reassuring.

BL	STV	LTV	Accels	Decels
			ht _____ bpm duration _____ sec	type _____ duration _____ sec depth _____ bpm

41. What is the most likely cause of this pattern (13.9)? _____

42. What actions would you take in response to this pattern?

   a.   do nothing

   b.   turn the woman

   c.   discontinue Pitocin®

   d.   increase IV fluids

   e.   observe the pattern

   f.   apply oxygen by mask

   g.   notify the midwife or doctor

   h.   perform a vaginal examination

   i.   take maternal blood pressure

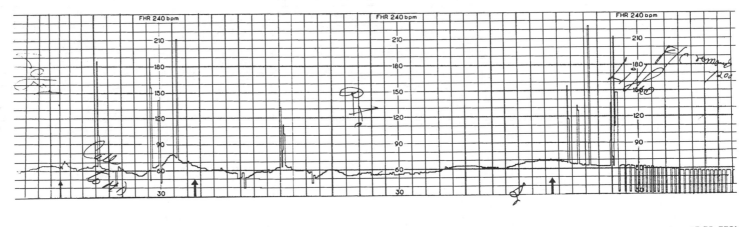

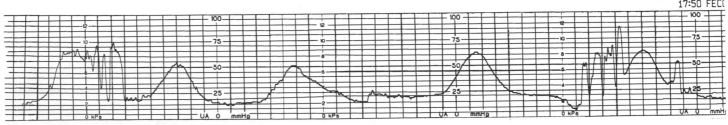

13.10 **Strip 10: This fetal heart rate pattern occurred within 7 minutes after the epidural test dose. The maternal blood pressure was 75/35.**

43. What 3 immediate actions would you take?

_____

_____

_____

44. If the FHR recovered to a rate greater than 160 bpm would the fetus be out of jeopardy? _____

45. Is the fetal heart rate adequate to perfuse the fetal brain? _____

ANSWERS

Answers To Strip Evaluation

Strip 1
1. 120-125
2. less than
3. 40-50
4. early

Strip 2
5. 25-90
6. 75-100
7. 20-50
8. variable

Strip 3
9. 25-45
10. 45-60
11. 40-45
12. late

Strip 4
13. 120-130
14. present
15. average
16. 145-150
17. 25-45
18. yes
19. no

Strip 5
20. episodic/nonperiodic
21. 5
22. 66 (this is European scale paper)
23. umbilical cord compression, uterine hyperstimulation

Strip 6

24. late
25. 1-4
26. 50-90
27. 75-100
28. 10-20
29. possible coupling at 0539-0540

Strip 7

30. 140-150
31. probably present, but this is an external ultrasound tracing
32. minimal to average
33. yes (see last minute)
34. no
35. no
36. LAHF waves or low amplitude high frequency waves or uterine irritability

Strip 8

37. 130-135 bpm (European scale paper), present STV, minimal LTV, no accels, only shoulders on variable decelerations, variable decels x 30 sec ⇓ 110-115 bpm
38. b
39. b, e, g if the pattern is unrelieved by your actions or she has a scarred uterus as variable decelerations are the most common deceleration pattern when the uterus is tearing (rupturing)

Strip 9

40. 125-140 bpm, 0 STV, 0 LTV, 0 accels, 0 decels
41. Demerol and uterine hyperstimulation with possible fetal hypoxia
42. b, c, d, e, f, g; remove oxygen once signs of fetal well-being return and the uterus is contracting normally

Strip 10

43. discontinue Pitocin®; call the surgeon, anesthesia provider, operating room crew, and pediatrician stat; provide an IV bolus of a non-glucose solution and Ephedrine® as ordered
44. no, that would be a rebound tachycardia which is highly unlikely with such profound bradycardia, suspect it's maternal heart rate doubling
45. no

A score of 40 correct is excellent. If you scored less than 40 correct, go back and reevaluate the images.

Now, let's look at how one group tried to reach consensus in the definitions of some fetal monitoring concepts in Section 14.

Section 14
NICHD Definitions

In the United States between May 1995 and November 1996, a National Institute of Child Health and Human Development (NICHD) panel composed of 17 physicians and 1 nurse met in Bethesda, Maryland and Chicago, Illinois. The group became known as the National Institutes of Health Research Planning Workshop. They were tasked with reaching consensus on recognition criteria of fetal monitoring concepts and to publish research recommendations for fetal heart rate (FHR) tracing analysis. Julian Parer, PhD, MD chaired the committee. He wrote that the purpose of the guidelines for nomenclature "was to achieve simplicity and brevity" (Parer, 1998, p. 560). Dr. Parer also explained that his committee believed that an FHR window of 10 minutes should be enough to see a baseline lasting at least 2 minutes and the baseline need not stay within any arbitrary range such as 110 to 150 bpm.

**NICHD
RESEARCH
GUIDELINES FOR
INTERPRETATION**

In 1997, the work of the NICHD panel produced definitions that were developed for visual interpretation of the FHR pattern whether or not an electrode or the external ultrasound was used to assess the FHR. Their definitions applied to both antepartal and intrapartal tracing analysis without any relationship to hypoxemia or metabolic acidosis (Electronic fetal heart, 1997a, 1997b).

The patterns were broadly differentiated into three categories: baseline, episodic, and periodic. In addition, gestational age was considered particularly when the panel described accelerations. They also felt the tracing should be evaluated in the context of the maternal medical condition, prior fetal assessment test results, and medications.

BASELINE

Baseline

This was defined as the approximate mean or average FHR rounded to increments of 5 beats per minute (bpm) during a 10 minute segment. The baseline excluded episodic or periodic changes, marked variability, and segments that differed by more than 25 bpm. The NICHD consensus group also decided that *at least 2 minutes* were needed in a 10 minute period to determine the baseline. However, if the baseline was not able to be determined, one would need to look back on the previous 10 minute segment or segments to determine the baseline. The group did not say if the 2 minutes needed to determine the baseline had to be consecutive.

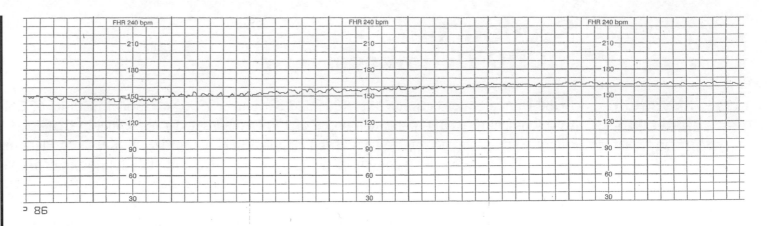

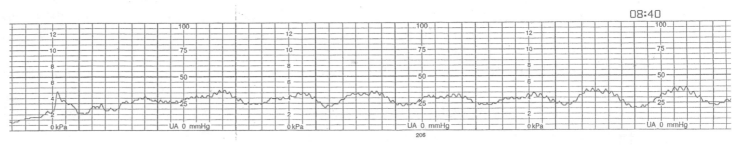

14.1   *Using the NICHD criteria, the baseline in this example would be rising from 150 to 155 to 165 if one uses increments of 5 bpm. Rising baseline was not a concept that was defined by the NICHD group.*

Bradycardia

The group decided fetal bradycardia would be a baseline less than 110 bpm. Using the NICHD descriptors to assess a baseline, one would need at least 2 minutes at less than 110 bpm to identify the baseline as bradycardic. They suggested that if the baseline were unstable that bradycardia may need to be quantitated by its actual FHR in bpm.

Tachycardia

The group decided fetal tachycardia would be a baseline greater than 160 bpm. Using the NICHD descriptors to assess a baseline, one would need at least 2 minutes at more than 160 bpm to identify the baseline as tachycardic. They suggested that if the baseline were unstable that tachycardia may need to be quantitated by its actual FHR in bpm.

Short-term Variability

Apparently the NICHD group could not reach consensus as to whether or not beat-to-beat variability or short-term variability could be interpretable to the unaided eye. They did agree it was quantifiable using the computer. Therefore, they never agreed STV was not a concept. The NICHD group felt that short-term variability was usually interpreted *with* long-term variability as "a unit."

Variability

Four categories were suggested by the NICHD group for categorizing baseline variability. According to the NICHD panel, to have variability, the baseline needs ***at least 2 or more cycles per minute***. Clearly, based on the visualization of cycles per minute, variability as defined by the NICHD panel is the same as the traditional long-term variability concept.

The four categories for variability suggested by the NICHD group are:

Absent: amplitude from peak to trough is undetectable
Minimal: amplitude from peak to trough more than undetectable and less than or equal to 5 bpm
Moderate: amplitude from peak to trough 6 to 25 bpm
Marked: amplitude from peak to trough more than 25 bpm.

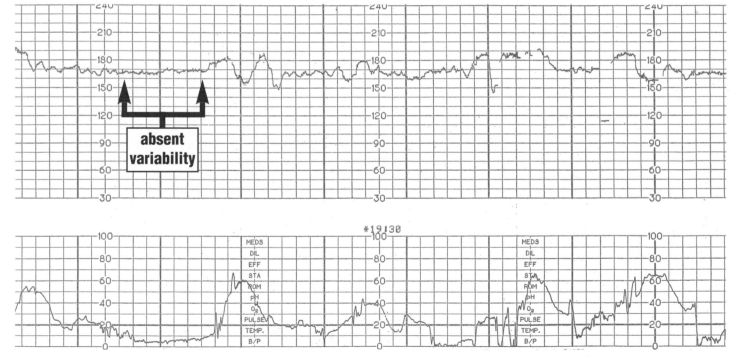

14.2 If variability is assessed as a unit, do you think short-term variability is also absent?

Sinusoidal Pattern

The NICHD group did not distinguish between pathologic sinusoidal (formerly true sinusoidal) patterns and benign or physiologic sinusoidal (formerly pseudosinusoidal) patterns. They defined a sinusoidal pattern as something distinct from a baseline and suggested that a sinusoidal pattern is a smooth, sine wave-like pattern of regular frequency and amplitude.

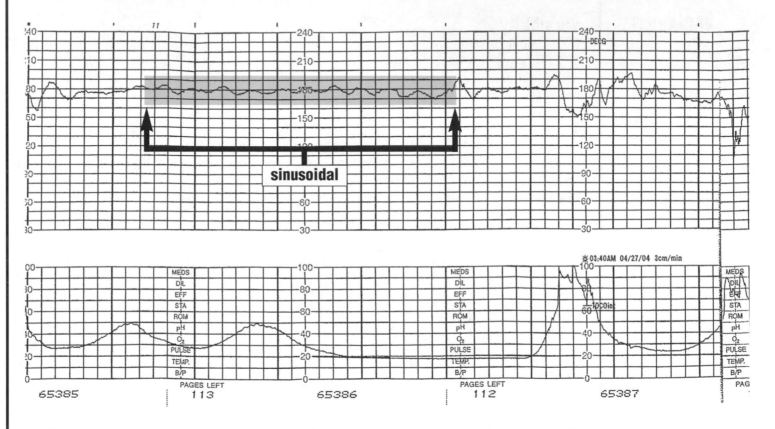

14.3 *This sinusoidal pattern was a pathologic pattern and occurred minutes before fetal decompensation to a terminal bradycardic level. The baby was born asphyxiated and has permanent brain damage. Note the tachycardic rate. Would you record "sinusoidal" or a baseline rate of 180 bpm? Recommendations for documentation of a sinusoidal pattern were not provided by the NICHD group.*

EPISODIC AND PERIODIC CHANGES

Episodic and Periodic Changes

Episodic changes are FHR patterns that do *not* occur in the presence of uterine contractions.

Periodic changes occur in the presence of uterine contractions.

Periodic and episodic changes might be abrupt or gradual, however, the NICHD committee failed to include the descriptor "episodic" or "periodic" in their definitions of accelerations and decelerations. In order to determine if a change is episodic or periodic, a good quality tracing for visual identification of these changes is helpful.

ACCELERATIONS

Accelerations

The NICHD group made no distinction between uniform and spontaneous accelerations. They defined an acceleration as an increase in the FHR above the baseline with an *abrupt* onset. The NICHD group felt the acceleration onset to peak time should be *less than 30 seconds*. They also made a distinction between fetuses at more than 32 weeks of gestation and less than 32 weeks of gestation. In the fetus at more than 32 weeks of gestation, the acme of the acceleration should be 15 or more bpm above the baseline to be called an acceleration. It also needed to last 15 or more seconds (see figure 14.4). In the less than 32 week gestation, the acceleration could have a peak 10 or more bpm above the baseline and last 10 or more seconds. The group had no recommendations for analysis of tracings of women who had no prenatal care and were in active labor with no time for an ultrasound or a determination of gestational age.

The NICHD group also suggested a new concept, i.e., prolonged acceleration. This was defined as an acceleration that lasted 2 or more minutes but less than 10 minutes in duration. If the acceleration lasted 10 or more minutes, they labeled it as a baseline change.

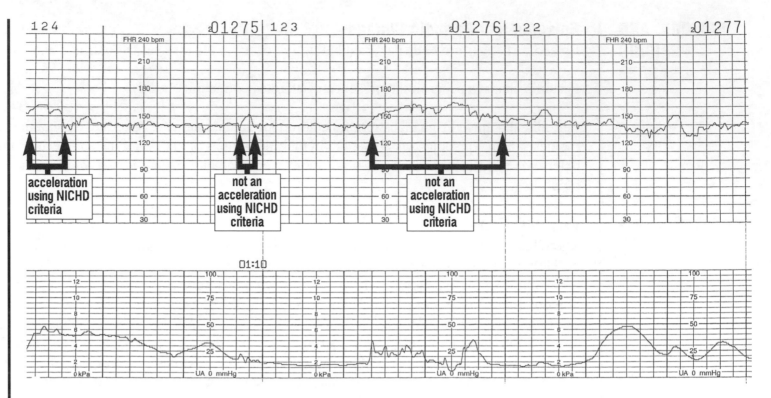

14.4 The NICHD criteria for an acceleration excludes some accelerations that also have meaning.

LATE DECELERATION

Late Deceleration

This was defined by the NICHD group as a visually apparent gradual decrease and gradual return to baseline associated with a uterine contraction. *Gradual was defined as lasting 30 or more seconds*. They suggested that the decrease in the FHR should be calculated from the most recently determined portion of the baseline and that the nadir of the deceleration occurred after the peak of the contraction. They decided that in most cases, the onset, nadir, and recovery of the late deceleration occurred after the beginning, peak, and end of the contraction (see figure 14.5).

EARLY DECELERATION

Early Deceleration

The group defined this type of deceleration as a *gradual decrease that took 30 or more seconds* to reach the nadir and it was associated with a contraction. They also felt that the return to baseline would be gradual (30 or more seconds). As with their definition of a late deceleration, the decrease in the FHR should be calculated from the most recently determined portion of the baseline. In the case of an early deceleration, the group decided that in most cases, the onset, nadir, and recovery of the deceleration was coincident with the onset, peak, and end of the contraction.

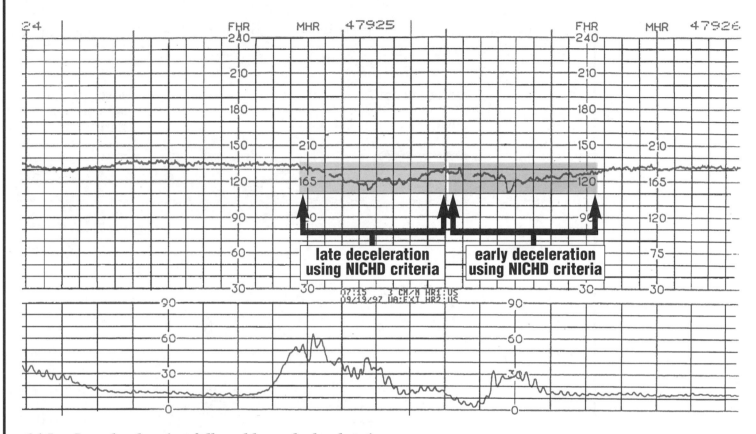

14.5   *Late deceleration followed by early deceleration.*

Variable Deceleration

According to the NICHD group, a variable deceleration is a visually apparent abrupt decrease in the FHR. Abrupt was defined as onset to nadir of *less than 30 seconds*. Like late and early decelerations, the decrease was based on the most recent portion of the baseline and had to be 15 or more bpm deep to be called a variable deceleration and it had to last 15 or more seconds but less than 2 minutes from its onset to its return to baseline.

In the traditional system, variable decelerations are described by their duration and depth. The NICHD group recognized that any deceleration could be quantitated by the depth of the nadir in bpm, excluding spikes or artifact and by the duration in seconds or minutes from its onset to end.

They suggested that recurrent decelerations occurred with 50 percent or more of the contractions in a 20 minute segment of the tracing.

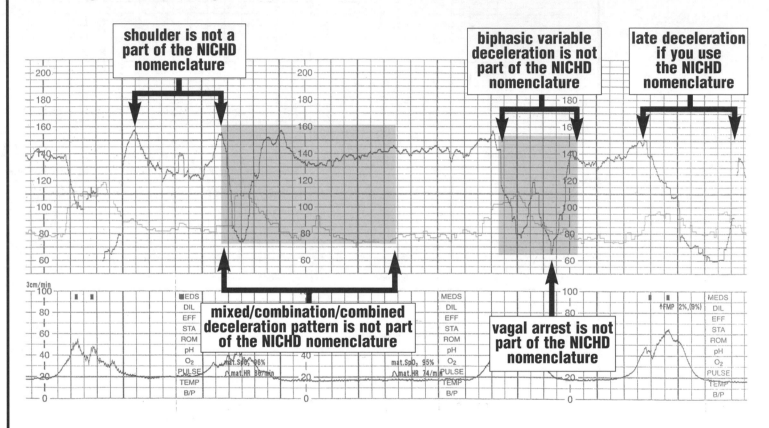

14.6   *Confusion has been reported by some clinicians when they saw only variable decelerations but where instructed to strictly apply the NICHD group's rule of 30 seconds or more to the nadir as a characteristic of late decelerations. The last deceleration is a severe variable deceleration using traditional terminology. Note this is European-scaled paper.*

Prolonged Deceleration

This was defined by the NICHD group as a visually apparent decrease in the FHR that was at *least 15 bpm deep* and lasted 2 or more minutes but less than 10 minutes from its onset to return to baseline.

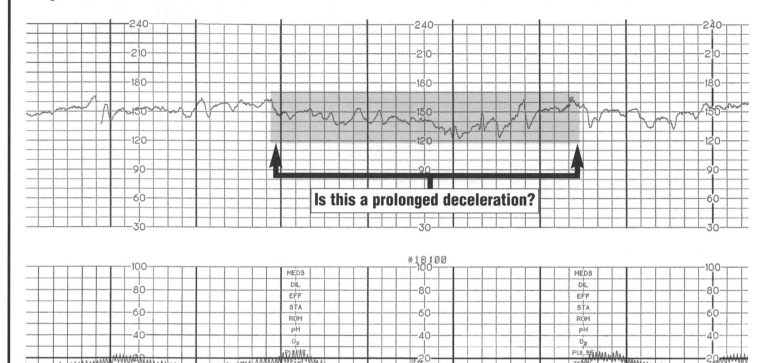

Is this a prolonged deceleration?

14.7   *If you decide the baseline is 150 bpm, this will not be a prolonged deceleration if you accept the NICHD group's criteria of a drop of at least 15 bpm for 2 or more minutes to call the deceleration prolonged.*

Limitations of the NICHD Nomenclature

The cognitive process of combining the assessment of short-term and long-term variability, i.e., assessing the two as one "unit" of variability has never been studied. Probably, it is best to teach each concept first. If clinicians are briefly at the bedside, they probably will scan the tracing and see less of the image, especially all of the component parts, than nurses or individuals who spend more time at the bedside. Those with more time to evaluate the tracing should be able to distinguish each component of the baseline, i.e., short-term and long-term variability (Murray, 1992).

The composition of the NICHD group included one nurse who was working at the time in a university hospital for the department of obstetrics and gynecology and 17 physicians, mostly from university obstetrics and gynecology departments. There was a representative from the National Institutes of Health on the committee as well. Based on the group's composition, it would only seem reasonable that their ideas should be tested first in an academic research setting, especially since community hospital-based nurses, certified nurse midwives, and obstetricians were not invited to participate. Thankfully, the NICHD group recognized that some of the definitions they proposed may be inadequate for bedside usage. Bedside clinicians do more than identify images. They add physiologic meaning which is critical to appropriately respond to the needs of the fetus. Since Dr. Parer (1998) wrote that the NICHD committee made no assumptions related to the cause of the patterns or their relationship to hypoxemia or metabolic acidemia, one needs to exercise caution when applying their definitions since only a small number of studies have now been completed that used the NICHD criteria.

LIMITED RESEARCH USING THE NICHD NOMENCLATURE

It is promising that researchers who used the NICHD nomenclature to identify features of the tracing during the two hours prior to delivery found a relationship between late decelerations, absent accelerations, and absent variability and umbilical artery blood gases (Sameshima et al., 2005a). In addition, they discovered a relationship between acute intrauterine infection, fetal tachycardia and cerebral palsy (Sameshima et al., 2005b). Specifically, Sameshima and his colleagues (2005a, 2005b) evaluated the tracings of 10,030 infants born between 1995 and 2000. They found:

1. **Late decelerations with 50% or more of the contractions, absent accelerations, and absent variability** were related to an abnormally low (less than 7.0) umbilical artery pH. Of the 5,522 women with "low-risk" pregnancies, 1.8% had this pattern during the last two hours of labor (2005a).
2. **A nonreassuring pattern occurred in 24% of pregnancies with an intrauterine infection** (2005b). Nonreassuring patterns included recurrent late decelerations (with 50% or more of the contractions), severe variable decelerations ["severe" is used in their report but was not defined by the NICHD], and prolonged decelerations.

It is interesting that they identified no fetuses with early decelerations in any of the tracings (Sameshima et al., 2005a). This suggests one of two possibilities:

1. Women studied did not have fetuses who exhibited head compression in the last two hours of labor or
2. The NICHD criteria was inadequate for researchers to distinguish early decelerations from late decelerations.

PEAK-TO-NADIR LAG TIME

What may be needed to enhance the NICHD definitions is the addition of the peak-to-nadir lag time recognition criteria. In the past, researchers found the contraction *peak to deceleration nadir lag time of early decelerations was usually less than 20 second*s, but 20 or more seconds for late decelerations (Myers et al. 1972, O'Gureck et al., 1972, Wood et al., 1969). Myers et al. (1972) found the average peak-to-nadir lag time for early decelerations was 3.5 seconds but 41 seconds for late decelerations and suggested that 18 seconds would be a good dividing time between the two. O'Gureck et al. (1972) found early decelerations had a lag time that is less than or equal to 20 seconds but the lag time of late decelerations was more than 20 seconds. Wood et al. (1969) reported the peak-to-nadir lag time of late decelerations was 18 or more seconds.

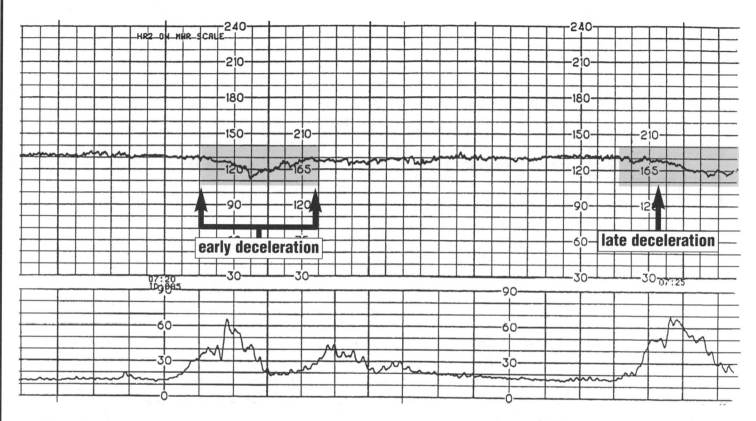

14.8   *The first deceleration would be classified as a late deceleration if you strictly apply the NICHD definitions since the onset to nadir is 30 seconds and the nadir occurs after the peak of the contraction. However, using the peak-to-nadir research findings, this would best be classified as an early deceleration. The second deceleration would best be classified as a late deceleration. It meets the NICHD criteria for 30 seconds to the nadir and also meets the traditional research finding of a peak-to-nadir lag time of more than 20 seconds.*

Tachycardia, Acute Chorioamnionitis and Cerebral Palsy

Samishema and his colleagues (2005b) used the NICHD nomenclature in their evaluation of the last two hours of the FHR pattern prior to delivery. They found that *when there was an acute intrauterine infection, cerebral palsy was related to fetal tachycardia* (odds ratio 11) *and/or a gestational age of less than 34 weeks* (odds ratio 9.4). An odds ratio is a statistic used in an analysis called logistic regression. It is the number of true positives multiplied by true negatives divided by the number of false positives multiplied by false negatives. Using these findings, the odds of the infant being diagnosed by the age of 2 with cerebral palsy when there was an acute intrauterine infection *and* fetal tachycardia was 11 times greater than if there was no fetal tachycardia. For many years, critics of fetal monitoring have suggested that there is no relationship between the fetal heart rate and cerebral palsy. This is perhaps the first research finding that has suggested there is a relationship between fetal tachycardia with acute chorioamnionitis within the two hours prior to delivery and cerebral palsy that was diagnosed by the age of 2.

No Improvement in Agreement in Interpretation Using NICHD Nomenclature

The NICHD group desired a study to determine intraobserver and interobserver agreement as measured by the kappa statistic and before and after instruction in their classification system to see if training in this system resulted in an improvement in agreement. Dr. Lawrence Devoe, who was a member of the NICHD consensus group, and his colleagues designed a study related to interobserver agreement (2000). They compared visual analyses of intrapartal FHR tracings according to the National Institute of Child Health and Human Development guidelines with the analyses by an automated FHR monitoring system. They conducted their study between May 1 and July 1, 1998. The visual analysis of 50 different 1 hour tracings at 10 minute intervals was compared with the analysis of a computer program (Hewlett-Packard TraceVue; HP GmbH, Böblingen, Germany). The tracings were evaluated by a registered nurse, a certified nurse midwife, an obstetrics resident physician, and a maternal-fetal medicine faculty member. When compared with the computer analysis of the tracings, the four clinicians had less than 63% agreement on the number of accelerations and 52% agreement on the number of decelerations. Agreement on the baseline rate (one number rounded to an increment of 5 bpm) was 83.5% to 88.1%. The authors concluded that the use of the NICHD guidelines for visual FHR analysis did not increase agreements on most FHR features beyond those expected by chance. They also suggested that computer analysis of tracings could eliminate interobserver variation.

Conclusion

Universal agreement on the recognition criteria, labels, categorization, and physiology related to interpretation of the FHR pattern is a noble but unobtainable goal. In addition, perfect agreement among clinicians or between clinicians and a software program is also unobtainable. Therefore, the best we can hope for is to acquire a broad and deep knowledge of fetal monitoring concepts so that we can properly identify each FHR pattern component and the fetal physiology it most likely represents so that we may promptly respond to the needs of the fetus.

REFERENCES

References

Devoe, L., Golde, S., Kilman, Y., Morton, D., Shea, K., & Waller, J. (August 2000). A comparison of visual analyses of intrapartum FHR tracings according to the new National Institute of Child Health and Human Development guidelines with computer analyses by an automated FHR monitoring system. *American Journal of Obstetrics and Gynecology, 183*(2), 361-366.

Electronic FHR monitoring: Research guidelines for interpretation. (1997a). *American Journal of Obstetrics and Gynecology, 177*, 1385-1390.

Electronic FHR monitoring: Research guidelines for interpretation. (1997b). *Journal of Obstetric, Gynecologic, and Neonatal Nursing, 26*, 635-640.

Murray, M. L. (1992). A comparison of fetal monitor concept learning from a learner-controlled versus teacher-controlled instructional strategy. (Doctoral Dissertation). Albuquerque. University of New Mexico.

Murray, M. L. (1997). *Antepartal and intrapartal fetal monitoring (2nd ed.).* Albuquerque, NM: Learning Resources International, Inc. www.fetalmonitoring.com.

Murray, M. L. (2006). *Antepartal and intrapartal fetal monitoring (3rd ed.).* Albuquerque, NM: Learning Resources International, Inc. www.fetalmonitoring.com.

Myers, G. G., Kraphol, A. J., Peterson, R. D., & Caldeyro-Barcia, R. (1972). New method for measuring lag time between human uterine contraction and the effect on the FHR. *American Journal of Obstetrics and Gynecology, 112*(1), 39-45.

O'Gureck, J. E., Roux, J. F., & Newman, M. R. (1972). A practical classification of FHR patterns. *Obstetrics and Gynecology, 40*(3), 356-361.

Parer, J. (August 1998). Reply to Bernades, J. & Perreira, A. C. Some concerns about the new research guidelines for interpretation of electronic FHR monitoring. [Letter]. *American Journal of Obstetrics and Gynecology, 179*(2), 560-561.

Samishema, H., & Ikenouc, T. (January 2005a). Predictive value of late decelerations for fetal acidemia in unselective low-risk pregnancies. *American Journal of Perinatology, 22*(1), 19-23.

Samishema, H., Ikenoue, T., Ikeda, T., Kamitomo, M., & Ibara, S. (May 2005b). Association of nonreassuring FHR patterns and subsequent cerebral palsy in pregnancies with intrauterine bacterial infection. *American Journal of Perinatology, 22*(4), 181-187.

Wood, C., Newman, W., Lumley, J., & Hammond, J. (1969). Classification of FHR in relation to fetal scalp blood measurements and Apgar score. *American Journal of Obstetrics and Gynecology, 105*(6), 942-948.

SECTION 15
Skills Validation

Name: _____

ID Number: _____

Date: _____

Skills Validation Sheet
for External Fetal Monitor Application

	Level
1. Positions woman to optimize fetal perfusion.	
2. Prior to application, inspects tocotransducer and ultrasound transducer for damage.	
3. Manually tests ultrasound transducer.	
4. Manually tests tocotransducer.	
5. Observes auto test or manually tests fetal monitor. Confirms monitor is properly printing and lighted display is complete.	
6. Performs Leopold's Maneuvers.	
7. Properly places tocotransducer on the abdomen based on fetal gestational age.	
8. Evaluates tracing quality and sets the uterine activity baseline as needed.	
9. Properly places ultrasound transducer over the fetal back.	
10. Evaluates tracing quality.	
11. Documents patient identification information on tracing.	
12. Verbalizes limitations of external fetal monitoring to instructor.	

Levels

I.   Hesitates, needs assistance to complete task

II. Requires verbal cues, motions fluid

III. Proceeds accurately and independently without cues

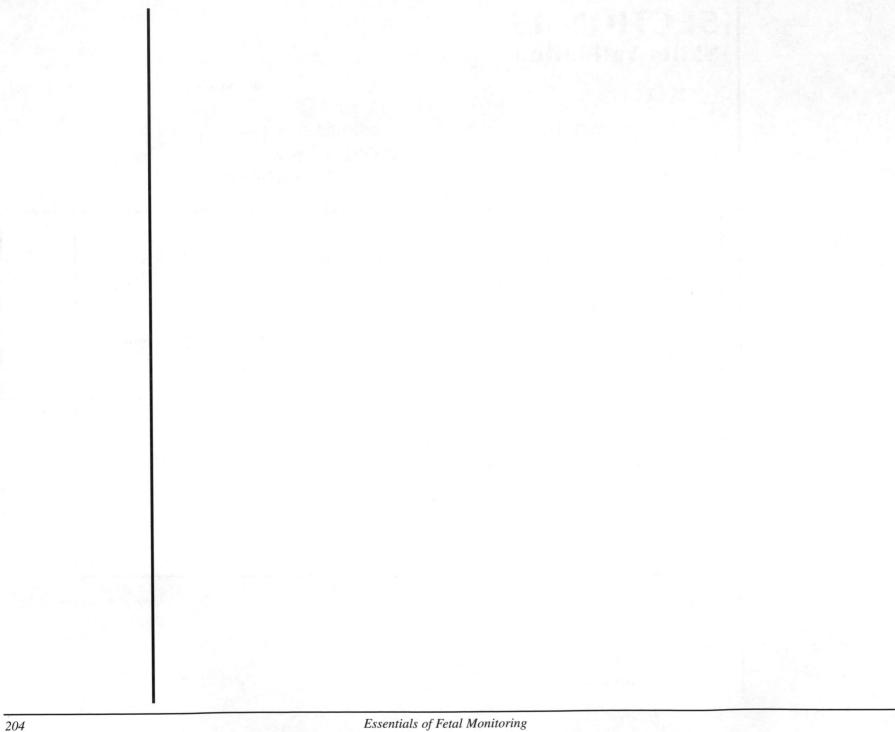

Skills Validation Sheet
for Auscultation of Fetal Heart Rate and Palpation of Uterine Activity

Level

1. Performs Leopold's Maneuvers to determine fetal lie and position of fetal back.	
2. Correctly uses and places fetoscope over fetal back.	
3. Listens with the fetoscope for 1 minute. In labor, listens before, during, and after a contraction.	
4. Determines fetal heart rate with fetoscope or hand-held doppler. If doppler is used, simultaneously determines maternal heart rate (pulse).	
5. Records signs of fetal well-being: • baseline; verbalizes normal range for gestational age • highest rate of audible acceleration(s) • deceleration(s) and lowest rate • palpates fetal movement.	
6. Palpates and records frequency, duration, strength, and relaxation of contractions.	

Levels

I. Hesitates, needs assistance to complete task

II. Requires verbal cues, motions fluid

III. Proceeds accurately and independently without cues

Name: _____

ID Number: _____

Date: _____

Troubleshooting EFM equipment

Level

• Verbalizes procedure to diminish gaps in the printed fetal heart rate or uterine activity tracing and protocol if the printout is too dark or too light.	
• Knows and can state procedure of when and where to send the monitor for repair.	

Levels

I.   Hesitates, needs assistance to complete task

II.   Requires verbal cues, motions fluid

III. Proceeds accurately and independently without cues

Name: _____

ID Number: _____

Date: _____

Spiral Electrode (SE) Application

Level

1. Verbalizes two risks and one benefit for SE use.	
2. Identifies fetal heart rate characteristics that indicate a need for a SE.	
3. Verbalizes placement locations.	
4. Organizes equipment prior to SE placement.	
5. Opens SE package.	
6. Dons sterile glove and applies lubricating gel.	
7. Identifies cervical dilatation and presenting part.	
8. Releases wires from wire lock.	
9. Retracts SE inside outer guide to protect vaginal wall prior to insertion.	
10. Inserts outer guide with retracted SE into vagina.	
11. Reverifies fetal presenting part.	
12. Advances outer guide until flush with presenting part.	
13. Advances SE.	
14. Rotates SE 180° clockwise.	
15. Attaches SE to SE cable.	
16. Evaluates quality of tracing.	
17. Inspects insertion site after delivery.	

Verification of Preceptor	Date	Pt ID Number
1. _____	_____	_____
2. _____	_____	_____
3. _____	_____	_____

Levels

I.   Hesitates, needs assistance to complete task

II.   Requires verbal cues, motions fluid

III. Proceeds accurately and independently, provides patient education, identifies interventions as needed based on tracing

Name: _____

ID Number: _____

Date: _____

Fetal Monitor Scavenger Hunt

Item	Location
1. Fetoscope	
2. Hand-held doppler	
3. Fetal monitor paper	
4. Fetal monitor belts	
5. Tocotransducer	
6. Ultrasound transducer	
7. Ultrasound coupling gel	
8. Spiral electrode	
9. Spiral electrode cable	
10. Intrauterine pressure catheter (IUPC) (read instructions on package, identify brand name)	
11. IUPC cable	
12. Maternal ECG cable for fetal monitor	
13. Electrodes for maternal ECG cable	
14. Maternal pulse oximeter finger probe and cable for fetal monitor	
15. Amniotomy hook	
16. Extra ultrasound transducer	

Item	Location
17. Extra tocotransducer	
18. IV tubing	
19. Blood tubing	
20. Fetal scalp blood sampling kit (if applicable)	
21. Cord blood gas kit or 1 ml syringe, heparin (1000 U/ml), ice basin or zip lock bags, and labels	
22. Policies and procedures related to fetal monitoring: • Nonstress test • Contraction stress test • Intrapartal fetal monitoring • Amnioinfusion • Other: _____ _____	

GLOSSARY OF FETAL HEART MONITORING TERMS

A

Ab: number of miscarriages (abortions) and births before 20 weeks' gestation, includes spontaneous (SAB) and therapeutic or elective abortions (TAB/EAB).

Abruptio placentae (placental abruption): premature separation of the placenta prior to delivery of the fetus.

Acceleration: an increase in the fetal heart rate above the baseline level. There are two types: uniform and spontaneous.

Acidemia: acid in the blood, specifically abnormal increase in hydrogen ion concentration due to the accumulation of an acid or a loss of base.

Acidosis: the abnormal accumulation of carbon dioxide (respiratory acidosis) or lactic acid (metabolic acidosis).

Agonal pattern: A bradycardic fetal heart rate of a decompensating fetus with a surge of catecholamines. An agonal pattern lacks short-term variability and is less than 100 beats per minute with upward and downward swings that last 20 or more seconds.

Amnioinfusion: instillation of an isotonic, glucose-free solution, such as normal saline or lactated Ringer's solution, into the uterus.

Amnion: inner membrane of the sac that encloses the fetus.

Amniotomy: breaking the bag of waters, the artificial rupture of fetal membranes (AROM).

Antepartal: before birth, pertaining to the period spanning conception to the onset of labor.

Anoxia: absence of oxygen within the tissues.

Apgar score: system of scoring neonate's physical condition one minute and five minutes after birth. The color or appearance (A), heart rate or pulse (P), response to stimuli or grimace (G), muscle tone or activity (A), and respirations (R) are assessed. Each can receive a maximum of 2 points. The maximum Apgar score is 10.

Arrhythmia: See dysrhythmia.

Artifact: irregularities on the monitor tracing due to poor reception of the fetal heart signal which appears as scattered dots, gaps on the tracing, or lines.

B

Asphyxia: a condition due to lack of oxygen resulting in impending or actual cessation of life, from Greek meaning "a stopping of the pulse." Implies a reduction in PO_2 (hypoxia), elevation of PCO_2 (hypercapnia), and lowering of blood pH and bicarbonate or mixed acidosis with respiratory and metabolic components. Asphyxia is preceded by anaerobic metabolism. Asphyxia can precede cell damage and/or death.

Auscultation: act of listening for sounds within the body; assisted by use of a stethoscope and/or fetoscope.

Ballotable head: A fetal head that has not descended into the pelvis, it floats up when touched.

Baroreceptors: Nerves that respond to changes in arterial diameter and blood pressure. Fetal baroreceptors that affect the fetal heart rate are found in the carotid sinuses and aorta. They are also known as stretch or pressor receptors.

Baseline (BL):   the fetal heart rate over a period of time, not including accelerations or decelerations. The BL may be recorded as a range or an average rate.

Beat-to-beat variability (BTBV):   The fluctuation or change in the interval between R waves or systole on the fetal electrocardiogram (ECG) measured in milliseconds (msec) by the fetal monitor. The average BTBV is 7.7 msec. When BTBV is present, short-term variability is also present.

Benign sinusoidal: A well-fetus pattern with $1^1/2$ or more cycles per minute resembling a pathologic sinusoidal pattern but preceded or followed by fetal movement and accelerations. Also called a physiologic sinusoidal pattern.

Bradycardia: a fetal heart rate less than 100 bpm (term and postterm) or less than 120 bpm (preterm).

C

Caput succedaneum: swelling occurring in and under the scalp of the fetus during labor after rupture of membranes. A localized pitting edema in the scalp of a fetus that may overlie sutures of the skull. It is usually formed during labor as a result of the circular pressure of the cervix on the fetal occiput.

Cervix (Cx):   neck of the uterus which protrudes into the vagina.

Chemoreceptors: pH, pO_2, and pCO_2 sensitive nerves that line the fourth ventricle near the brainstem and are also found in the aortic and carotid bodies. They respond to changes in pH in the cerebral spinal fluid and pH, PO_2 and PCO_2 in arterial blood.

Compensatory pattern: A classification of a fetal heart rate pattern indicating fetal hypoxia, hypovolemia, hypotension or hypertension. Examples include tachycardia with spontaneous accelerations, end-stage bradycardia with accelerations, a saltatory pattern or marked long-term variability, one prolonged deceleration, accelerations with late decelerations. Compensatory patterns always have accelerations and short-term variability.

Contraction stress test (CST): antepartum surveillance method using induced or spontaneous contractions to evaluate fetal oxygen reserves and placental function. Induced contractions may be from endogenous or exogenous oxytocin.

Cycle: also called a sine wave, oscillation, or complex, the fluctuation of the fetal heart rate above, through and back to the average baseline level.

D

Deceleration: a distinct decrease in the FHR with a return to a baseline with a duration of less than 10 minutes. Decelerations are classified by their shape and/or timing in relation to uterine contractions.

Dilatation: expansion of the opening of the cervix from 1 to 10 cm.

Dip: A drop in the fetal heart rate below the baseline, often before or after a spontaneous acceleration. A dip may have a V shape and be less than 15 seconds in duration. A dip immediately following an acceleration may be a V or U shape and last longer than 15 seconds. A dip is innocuous. Preterm fetuses dip more than term or postterm fetuses.

Doppler ultrasound: instrument that emits and receives sound waves to determine the fetal heart rate.

Dysrhythmia: any variation from the normal rhythm of the heart.

E

Early deceleration: a deceleration of the fetal heart rate which is caused by compression of the fetal head and characterized by a gradual onset at the beginning of a contraction and a gradual offset or recovery to the baseline soon after the contraction ends. The nadir is < 18 seconds after the contraction peak.

EDD/EDC: expected date of delivery or confinement or due date calculated from the first day of the last menstrual period or estimated by other clinical parameters such as ultrasound measurements of the fetus.

Effacement: shortening or thinning of the cervical canal, usually during the early phase of dilatation, estimated by a percent. For example, 80% effaced indicates the cervix is approximately 4/5th of its original length. The closed cervix is 2.5 to 3 cm long.

Electronic fetal monitor (EFM): computer with paper printout used to show graphically and continuously the relationship between maternal uterine activity and the FHR.

End-stage bradycardia: Also called second-stage bradycardia with a 15 to 30 beats per minute drop from the fetal heart rate baseline level during the second stage of labor when the woman is pushing.

Engagement of the vertex occurs when the biparietal diameter has passed through the pelvic inlet and is clinically diagnosed when the leading bony portion of the fetal head is at or below the level of the ischial spines (station 0 or more)

Epidural: regional anesthesia administered through the back between L3 and L4 via a thin catheter in the epidural space outside of the spinal canal or the dura mater.

Extrinsic factors: Factors outside of the fetus that can affect the fetal heart rate, e.g., cord compression, placental abruption, maternal cardiac or oxygen problems.

F

Fetal distress: An ill-defined term suggesting the fetus has a high risk of asphyxia that can cause fetal brain damage if the asphyxial insult is not relieved. The term should not be used in clinical practice or documentation. Instead, nonreassuring fetus status should be used.

Fetal heart rate (FHR): fetal ventricular rate in beats per minute.

Fetal scalp electrode: see spiral electrode.

Fetal well-being: A nonhypoxic fetus who moves, usually just prior to or during an acceleration, and who has short-term variability and no decelerations.

Fundus: portion of the uterus which lies above the insertion of the fallopian tubes at the top of the uterus. The portion farthest from the mouth of an organ.

G

Gestation: time from conception to birth.

Gestational age: age of the embryo or fetus computed from the first day of the last menstrual period to the present, usually expressed in weeks.

Gravida (G): number of pregnancies.

H

Hematoma: localized collection of blood, usually clotted, caused by a break in the wall of a blood vessel.

Hyperstimulation: Also called tachysystole or hypercontractility. Contraction frequency is less than every two minutes with the contraction interval less than 60 seconds.

Hypertonus: Abnormally high resting tone or when the uterus is firm to palpation between contractions.

Hypoxemia: low blood oxygen content.

Hypoxia: deficiency of oxygen in the cells.

I

Intensity: when an intrauterine pressure catheter is in the uterus, the peak intrauterine pressure minus the resting tone.

Intrapartal: the period of time during labor and birth.

Intrauterine pressure catheter (IUPC): a fluid-filled or solid catheter inserted transvaginally into the uterus. Intrauterine pressure is conducted through the catheter, exerted on a pressure transducer, and transformed to an electronic signal, then printed on the tracing.

Intrinsic factors: Factors within the fetus that can affect the fetal heart rate, e.g., chemoreceptors, baroreceptors, catecholamines, adenosine, arginine vasopressin, the sympathetic nerves, and the vagus nerves or vagi.

Introitus: entrance to the vagina.

Ischial spines: the shortest diameter of the pelvis. Two prominent, palpable bony prominences.

L

Late deceleration: a deceleration of the fetal heart rate caused by uteroplacental insufficiency (low oxygen delivery) and characterized by a gradual, slanted onset after the contraction begins, and *usually* a slow return to baseline. The nadir is always 18 or more seconds after the contraction peak. Late decelerations tend to be similar in shape. They return to baseline after the contraction ends.

Long-term variability (LTV): the fluctuation of the fetal heart rate above and below an average baseline rate, LTV is evaluated each minute of the baseline by measuring the band-width of the baseline when there are 2 or more cycles per minute.

M

Low amplitude high frequency (LAHF) waves: Also called uterine irritability. The uterine activity waveform shows waves less than 30 seconds in duration with a less than 15 second interval. This is commonly associated with abruption, preterm labor, infection, or ketonuria due to dehydration.

Meconium: dark-green mucilaginous material in the intestine of the fetus. The normal contents of the baby's intestines, i.e., 80% water, 20% mucoproteins, mucopolysaccharides, and biliverdin.

Membranes: the sac surrounding the fetus.

Molding: shaping of the fetal head in adjustment to the size and shape of the pelvis and birth canal.

Midforceps: The application of forceps when the head is engaged but the leading point of the skull is above station +2. Application of forceps above station +2 may be attempted while simultaneously initiating preparations for a cesarean delivery in the event that the forceps maneuver is unsuccessful.

Montevideo units: from Uruguay, invented by Drs. Caldeyro-Barcia and Alvarez. The sum of the active pressure (peak minus resting tone) of contractions in a ten minute period.

Multipara: a woman who has completed two or more pregnancies to the stage of viability.

N

Nadir: Lowest point of a deceleration.

Nonperiodic (pattern): decelerations not related to contractions.

Nonreassuring pattern: A fetal heart rate pattern reflecting a deteriorating fetal status due to hypoxia and the continuing depletion of oxygen reserves which increase the risk of metabolic acidosis. Short-term variability may be absent. Accelerations are absent. There may be decelerations or a pathologic sinusoidal pattern.

Nonstress test (NST): antepartum surveillance method used to evaluate fetal condition by evaluation of the fetal heart rate pattern. An oxygenated, nonacidotic term fetus should have at least 2 accelerations in a 20 minute period with each acceleration peaking 15 bpm above the baseline and lasting 15 or more seconds at its base.

O

Occiput: back part of the head.

Ominous pattern: A fetal heart rate pattern associated with a fetus who has metabolic acidosis or asphyxia requiring immediate delivery. Accelerations and short-term variability are absent. Decelerations, terminal bradycardia, an agonal pattern, or a wandering baseline may be present. Ominous patterns are associated with fetal or neonatal death or poor neonatal outcomes.

Outlet forceps: The application of forceps when a) the scalp is visible at the introitus without separating the labia, b) the fetal skull has reached the pelvic floor, c) the sagittal suture is in the anterior-posterior diameter or in the right or left occiput anterior or posterior position, and d) the fetal head is at or on the perineum.

Overshoot: See variable deceleration.

Oxytocic: agent which acts like the naturally occurring hormone oxytocin, and stimulates contractions of the pregnant uterus.

Oxytocin Challenge Test (OCT): a CST which is conducted by stimulation of uterine contractions with intravenously administered oxytocin. NST criteria also apply to the CST, i.e., a well fetus has a reactive negative test.

Para (P) or parity: The number of fetuses delivered who were at least 500 grams or who had a gestational age of 20 weeks. Past obstetric history may be summarized in a series of numbers connected by hyphens. For example, pregnancies (gravida), term infants, premature infants, abortions, number of children currently alive may appear on the prenatal record as 3-2-1-0-3.

Paracervical block: local anesthesia injected around the cervix to relieve the pain of uterine contractions.

Parasympathetic nerves: Includes the 10th cranial nerve or the vagus. The right vagal branch innervates the sinoatrial node and the left vagal branch innervates the atrioventricular node. Vagal stimulation precedes decelerations, bradycardia, and creates short-term variability and a sawtooth pattern.

Periodic pattern: decelerations occurring in relation to contractions.

Pathologic sinusoidal pattern: An undulating baseline with $1^{1}/_{2}$ to 5 cycles per minute associated with fetal hypoxia, acidosis, and asphyxia. Hypoxia may be associated with severe fetal anemia with a hematocrit less than 20% and the compensatory release of arginine vasopressin from the posterior pituitary gland. Short-term variability will be decreased if the fetus is hypoxic but absent if the fetus is metabolically acidotic or asphyxiated. Fetal movement is decreased or absent. Accelerations are absent.

P

	Pattern:	the fetal heart rate plotted on heat sensitive paper in an electronic fetal heart monitor; including baseline rate, variability, accelerations, and decelerations.
	Placenta previa:	placenta lying partially or totally over the cervical os or opening.
	Position:	the relation of the presenting part, eg., fetal head or buttocks, to the maternal pelvis.
	Presentation:	the part of the baby that is over the birth canal.
	Presenting part:	portion of the fetus which is touched by the gloved examining finger(s) during a vaginal examination. The part of the fetus that is first into the birth canal.
	Primigravida:	a women pregnant for the first time.
	Primipara:	a woman who has delivered one fetus weighing 500 or more grams or who was 20 or more weeks of gestation when she delivered.
	Prolonged deceleration:	a nonperiodic deceleration characterized by a drop in the fetal heart rate that lasts at least 2 minutes but less than 10 minutes.
	Prostaglandins:	hormone-like unsaturated fatty acids that have an effect on blood vessels, smooth muscles, platelets, endocrine glands, the uterus, and the nervous system.
	Pseudosinusoidal:	See benign sinusoidal pattern.
R	**Reactive:**	An adjective to describe an acceleration that increases 15 beats per minute above the middle of the baseline and lasts 15 seconds at its base. Also a classification term for a nonstress test, or a contraction stress test (CST) that has two reactive accelerations in a 20 minute period, e.g., reactive negative CST.
	Reactivity:	A vague term with multiple definitions that is not recommended for use.
	Reassuring pattern:	A fetal heart rate pattern of a nonhypoxic fetus which has spontaneous accelerations and short-term variability. Fetal movement is present.
S	**Sawtooth pattern:**	Small baseline fetal heart rate fluctuations of 20 or more each minute resembling "little teeth" due to stimulation of the vagus in conjunction with stimulation of respiratory nerves in the brainstem. Reflects a fetal respiratory sinus dysrhythmia.
	Short-term variability (STV):	the consecutive beats per minute (bpm) rates plotted on moving fetal monitor paper, which appears as bumps, squiggles or even small lines 9 to 10 bpm long. STV is determined from beat-to-beat variability (BTBV).

	Sinusoidal pattern:	See pathologic sinusoidal pattern and benign sinusoidal pattern.
	Spiral electrode:	usually a stainless steel curved wire which is inserted under the fetal skin of the presenting part. It transmits the fetal heart electric current to the fetal monitor.
	Station:	the level (in centimeters) of the presenting part in relation to the ischial spines. (-) is above the spines, "O" is at the spines, and (+) is below the spines. If the fetal head (vertex) is presenting, station is the relationship of the estimated distance, in centimeters, between the bony portion of the fetal head and the level of the maternal ischial spines.
	Sympathetic nerves:	Nerves in the autonomic nervous system. When activated, the fetal heart rate increases. There will be accelerations, a rising baseline, or tachycardia.
T	**Tachycardia:**	in the fetus, a heart rate above 160 bpm. Maternal tachycardia is a rate above 100 bpm.
	Tocodynamometer/tocotransducer (TOCO):	pressure sensing device applied externally to the maternal abdomen to assess uterine contractions.
	Tonus or resting tone:	partial contraction of the uterine muscle between contractions, measured in mm Hg by an intrauterine pressure catheter or assessed by palpation.
	Tracing:	the paper and pattern of the fetal heart rate and/or contractions produced by an electronic fetal monitor. Also called a strip or strip chart.
	Transducer:	a device which senses a signal for conversion to an electronic form.
	True sinusoidal pattern:	See pathologic sinusoidal pattern.
U	**Uterine contractions (UC):**	periodic increase in intrauterine pressure. When externally palpated, uterine contractions are classified as mild, moderate, and strong.
	Uterine irritability:	See low amplitude high frequency waves.
	Uterine resting tone:	see tonus or resting tone.
	Uteroplacental reserve:	the amount of blood and oxygen available to support the fetus during contractions.
	Uteroplacental insufficiency:	an inadequate flow of oxygen from the intervillous space to the fetus, resulting in fetal hypoxemia.

V

Variability (FHRV): fetal heart rate variability has two components: long-term variability (the slow rhythmic fluctuations above and below an average baseline rate) and short-term variability which are instantaneous fluctuations in the fetal heart rate. The combination of these two types of variability reflects the interaction between parasympathetic and sympathetic branches of the central nervous system.

Variable deceleration: a deceleration of the fetal heart rate caused by umbilical cord compression and/or head compression (especially in the second stage of labor with pushing), characterized by a rapid onset and return to baseline, and a variable relationship to the contraction (may occur at any time during or between contractions). Variable decelerations may be preceded or followed by acceleratory phases, or shoulders.

Shoulders: brief increases in the fetal heart rate (usually less than 20 seconds in duration) that precede and follow a variable deceleration in response to umbilical vein compression. Shoulders are a compensatory sign and a part of the deceleration.

Overshoot: immediately following a variable deceleration, a high increase (> 20 bpm above the baseline) or a long increase (> 20 seconds in duration). Neither a shoulder nor an overshoot is classified as an acceleration. Rather, this acceleratory phase suggests a fetal response to hypoxia with release of catecholamines. Overshoots are a nonreassuring sign.

Variation: computer-generated analysis of the fetal heart rate over 1/16th of a minute (short-term variation) and each minute (long-term variation). Variation is calculated in milliseconds and is determined with an ultrasound transducer in place using specialized computer software.

Viable: a reasonable potential for survival if the fetus were delivered. In determining parity, viability is considered to be 500 grams or 20 weeks' gestation. However, a fetus will not survive if it is born at 20 weeks of gestation. A reasonable potential for survival appears to be delivery at 23 or more weeks' gestation, if neonatal intensive care facilities are available.

SUGGESTED ABBREVIATIONS

A

a	arterial
AB or ab	abortion
Abd	abdomen
ABG	arterial blood gases
accel(s)	acceleration(s)
ACTH	adrenocorticotropic hormone
adm	admission
A/G ratio	albumin/globulin ratio test
AFP	alpha fetoprotein
AGA	appropriate for gestational age
$AgNO_3$	silver nitrate
alb	albumin
AMA	against medical advice
amb	ambulate or ambulatory
amnio	amniocentesis
amt	amount
ANA	antinuclear antibodies
Angio	angiocath (intravenous catheter brand)
AO	aorta
AP	apical pulse
A-P	anterior/posterior
ARDS	Adult Respiratory Distress Syndrome
AROM	artificial rupture of membranes
ASA	acetylsalicylic acid (aspirin)
ASAP	as soon as possible
AV	Atrioventricular
ax	axilla

B

BBOW	bulging bag of water
b.i.d.	twice a day
BL	baseline
BM	bowel movement
BOW	bag of water
BP	blood pressure
BPM or bpm	beats per minute
BPP	biophysical profile

BR	bathroom
BTL	bottle
BUN	blood urea nitrogen

C

C	Centigrade/celsius
°C	degrees Celcius
CAN	cord around neck (nuchal cord)
CBC	complete blood count
CBG	capillary blood gases
cc	cubic centimeter(s)
cm	centimeter(s)
CO	carbon monoxide
CO_2	carbon dioxide
COHb or HbCO	carboxyhemoglobin
CPAP	continuous positive airway pressure
CPD	cephalopelvic disproportion
CPK	creatinine phosphokinase
CPR	cardiopulmonary resuscitation
CRP	C-reactive protein
C/S, C-Section	cesarean section
CSF	cerebrospinal fluid
CST	contraction stress test
CTX or UCs	contraction(s)/uterine contractions
CV	cardiovascular
CVA	cerebrovascular accident
CVP	central venous pressure
CX, cx	cervix

D

D_5LR	5% dextrose in lactated Ringer's (solution)
2,3-DPG	2, 3-diphosphoglycerate)
D	delta (Gk) representing change or difference
DAT	diet as tolerated
DC	discontinue
DC'd or dc'd	discontinued

decel(s)	deceleration(s)
del	delivery
decr or ↓	decrease
DFM	decreased fetal movement
DI	diabetes insipidus
DIC	disseminated intravascular coagulation or coagulopathy
Dig	digoxin
dil	dilatation
Disch	discharge
dk	dark
DKA	diabetic ketoacidosis
DM	diabetes mellitus
DNA	do not announce
DOB	date of birth
DR	delivery Room
Dr.	doctor
drsg	dressing(s)
DX or Dx	diagnosis

E

early decel(s)	early deceleration(s)
EBL	estimated blood loss
EBOW	evident bag of water
ECG	electrocardiogram
Echo	echocardiogram
EDC	estimated date of confinement (see EDD)
EDD	estimated date delivery/estimated due date
EDH	epidural hematoma
EEG	electroencephalogram
EENT	eyes, ears, nose and throat
EF	ejection fraction
EFM	electronic fetal monitoring
EFW	estimated fetal weight
EGA	estimated gestational age
ENT	Ears, nose and throat
epis	episiotomy
Eq	equivalent(s)
est	estimate or estimated
ETA	estimated time of arrival
ER	emergency room

ETT	endotracheal tube
exam	examination
Ext	external

F

F	fetal
FBS	fasting blood sugar
FA	fetus active
FAS	fetal accoustic stimulator
FBM	fetal breathing movements
FD	fetal demise (see IUFD for intrauterine fetal demise)
FDP	fibrinogen degradation products
Fe	iron
FECG	fetal electrocardiogram
FF or ff	fundus firm
FFP	fresh frozen plasma
FHR	fetal heart rate
FHT	fetal heart tones
F^IO_2	fractional inspired oxygen
fld	fluid
FM	fetal movement
FOB	father of baby
FP	fundal pressure
FSE	fetal scalp electrode (more appropriately abbreviated SE as it is only applied to the fetus)
FSH	follicle-stimulating hormone
FT	fingertip
F/U	fundus at umbilicus
FUO	fever of undetermined origin
Fx	fracture

G

g or gm	gram(s)
G	gravida
GA	gestational age
GBM	gross body movement(s)
GEST	gestation
G T P A L	gravida, term, preterm, aborta, living children

GTT	glucose tolerance test
gtt	drop(s)
GU	genitourinary
GYN	gynecology

H

h. or hr.	hour(s)
HA	headache
Hb or hgb	hemoglobin
HbA	adult hemoglobin
HbA_{1C}	hemoglobin A_{1C} (glycosylated hemoglobin)
HbF	fetal hemoglobin
HBP or HTN	high blood pressure/hypertension
HB_SA_g	hepatitis B surface antigen
HCT or hct	hematocrit
HCVD	hypertensive cardiovascular disease
HDL	high density lipoprotein
HEENT	Head, eyes, ears, nose and throat
HELLP	hemolysis, elevated liver enzymes, low platelets
HFD	high forceps delivery
H & H	hemoglobin and hematocrit
HL	heparin lock
H_2O	water
HOB	head of bed
Hosp	hospital
H & P	history and physical
hs	at bedtime
ht	height
HTN	hypertension
HTVD	hypertensive vascular disease
HX or Hx	history

I

I	iodine
IASD	Intra-atrial septal defect
IBOW	intact bag of water
IBW	ideal body weight
ICA	internal carotid artery
ICH	intracranial hemorrhage
ict	icterus

ICU	intensive care unit
I & D	incision and drainage
IDM	infant of diabetic mother
IG	immune globulin
incr or ↑	increase
Ind or ind	induction of labor
inf	infection
inj	inject(ion)
IU	International Unit (of hormone activity)
IUFD	intrauterine fetal demise
IUGR	intrauterine growth restriction, formerly intrauterine growth retardation
IUPC	intrauterine pressure catheter
IV	intravenous
IVAC	volume infusion pump
IVH	intraventricular hemorrhage
IVPB	intravenous piggyback
IVSD	intraventricular septal defect

K

K	potassium
K-B	Kleihauer-Betke test
KCL	potassium chloride
Kg or kg	kilogram
kPa	kilopascal (1 kPa = 7.5 mm Hg)

L

L or l	liter
lab	laboratory
lac	laceration
lap	laparotomy
lat	lateral
late decel(s)	late deceleration(s)
lb.	pound
LBP	low back pain
LBW	low birth weight
LC	living child
LDH	lactic dehydrogenase
LDRP	labor, delivery, recovery, post partum

LFD	low forcep delivery		MgSO$_4$	magnesium sulfate
lg	large		MHR	maternal heart rate
LGA	large for gestational age		MI	myocardial infarction
liq	liquid		midnoc	midnight
LLQ	left lower quadrant		min	minute
LMP	last menstrual period		ML	midline
LPM	liters per minute or liters by mask		ml	milliliter
L → R	left to right		MLE	midline episiotomy
L/S	lecithin/sphingomyelin ratio		mm	millimeter
LTV	long-term veriability		mm Hg	millimeters of mercury (1 mm Hg = 0.133 kPa)
LTV abs/LTV O	long-term variability absent (0-2 bpm BL bandwidth)		mmol	millimole
LTV min/LTV ↓	long-term variability minimal (3-5 bpm BL bandwidth)		MO	mineral Oil
LTV av	long-term variability average (6-10 bpm BL bandwidth)		MOM	milk of magnesia
			mo(s)	month(s)
			mosm	milliosmole
LTV mod/LTV ↑	long-term variability moderate (11-25 bpm BL bandwidth)		MPV	mean platelet volume
			MSF	meconium-stained fluid
LTV marked	long-term variability marked or saltatory (> 25 bpm bandwidth)		mU	milliunits
			mU/min	milliunits per minute
LOA	Left occiput anterior			
LOP	left occiput posterior			
LR	lactated Ringer's (solution)		**N**	
L-spine	lumbar spine		N	number
L	left		NB	newborn
LUOQ	left upper outer quadrant		NICU	neonatal intensive care unit
LUQ	left upper quadrant		NKA	no known allergies
lytes	electrolytes		NSVD	normal spontaneous vaginal delivery
			NST	nonstress test
			NSY	nursery
M			N/V	nausea and vomiting
mat	maternal			
max	maximum			
mcg	microgram (also µg)		**O**	
MCH	mean corpuscular hemoglobin		O$_2$	oxygen
MCHC	mean corpuscular hemoglobin concentration		OA	occiput anterior
			OB	obstetrics
MCV	mean corpuscular volume		OBRR	obstetrics recovery room
mec	meconium		OCT	oxytocin challenge test
mEq(s)	milliequivalent(s)		OP	occiput posterior
MFD	midforceps delivery		OT	occiput transverse
mg	milligram			
mg%	milligrams percent			

Basic Concepts in Antepartal and Intrapartal Fetal Monitoring

P

p	probability
P	partial pressure, eg. PO_2 is the partial pressure of oxygen
PAC	premature atrial contractions
PP	post partum
P_{50}	point on partial pressure axis on oxyhemoglobin dissociation curve of 50% hemoglobin saturation
PGE_2	prostaglandin E_2
PIGI	pregnancy-induced glucose intolerance
PIH	pregnancy-induced hypertension
PNV	postnatal visit
prolonged decel	prolonged deceleration
PP	post partum
PPROM	preterm premature rupture of membranes
PTL	postpartal tubal ligation
PROM	premature rupture of membranes
pt	patient

Q

q	every
Q	blood flow

R

RBCs	red blood cells
R/CS	repeat cesarean section
ROM	rupture of membranes
R → L	right to left
RR	recovery room

S

S	saturation, as in SaO_2
SE	spiral electrode
SGA	small for gestational age
SIDS	sudden infant death syndrome
SKB	single, keeping baby
SNKB	single, not keeping baby

spont	spontaneous
SROM	spontaneous rupture of membranes
S/S	signs and symptoms
S → S	side to side
STAT	immediately
STDs	sexually transmitted diseases
STV	short-term variability
STV +	short-term variability present
STV 0	short-term variability absent
STV inter	short-term variability intermittent
SVE	sterile vaginal examination
SVT	supraventricular tachycardia

T

TAB	therapeutic abortion
ThAB	threatened abortion
T/L	tubal ligation
TOCO or toco	tocodynamometer, tocotransducer
TOL	trial of labor
TOLAC	trial of labor after cesarean

U

UAC	umbilical artery catheter
UCs	uterine contractions
US	ultrasound (external monitoring)
UVC	umbilical venous catheter

V

vag	vaginal
var decel(s)	variable decelerations
VBAC	vaginal birth after cesarean section
VE	vaginal examination
VTX or vtx	vertex
VO_2	oxygen delivery (or oxygen consumption)

W, X, Y, Z

WNL	within normal limits
wt	weight
xylo	xylocaine
YOB	year of birth

Basic Concepts in Antepartal and Intrapartal Fetal Monitoring